Pocket Examiner in
Pathology

Pocket Examiner in
Pathology

P. N. Cowen BSc, PhD, MB, BS, FRCPath

Senior Lecturer in Pathology, University of Leeds; Honorary Consultant Pathologist, General Infirmary, Leeds, UK

F. G. Smiddy, MD, ChM, FRCS

Consultant Surgeon, General Infirmary, Leeds and Clayton Hospital, Wakefield, UK; Examiner in Pathology, College of Surgeons of England; Member of the Court of Examiners of the Royal College of Surgeons of England

Churchill Livingstone
EDINBURGH LONDON MELBOURNE AND NEW YORK 1986

Churchill Livingstone
Medical Division of Longman Group UK Limited

Distributed in the United States of America by Churchill Livingstone Inc., 1560 Broadway, New York, N.Y. 10036, and by associated companies, branches and representatives throughout the world.

© P. N. Cowen and F. G. Smiddy 1986

All rights reserved. No part of this publication may be reproduced, stored in a retrieval system, or transmitted in any form or by any means, electronic, mechanical, photocopying, recording or otherwise, without the prior permission of the publishers (Churchill Livingstone, Robert Stevenson House, 1–3 Baxter's Place, Leith Walk, Edinburgh EH1 3AF).

First published 1986

ISBN 0-443-03727-2

British Library Cataloguing in Publication Data
Cowen, P. N.
Pocket examiner in pathology.
1. Pathology—Problems, exercises, etc.
I. Title II. Smiddy, F. G.
616.07'076 RB119

Produced by Longman Singapore Publishers (Pte) Ltd.
Printed in Singapore

Preface

The subject of this Pocket Examiner must of necessity be dealt with in rather a truncated manner since answers to pathology essay questions are much longer than can be eased into the limited space available. Thus not only is there a constraint on the number of questions but also on the length of the answers. Nevertheless, it is hoped that by considering the topics of major importance which are dealt with, the student will either have his memory jogged, be edified or have his curiosity sufficiently aroused to encourage him to refer to a textbook. In the last respect, the authors feel that several good texts exist for further reference and would recommend, among others, *Muir's Textbook of Pathology* and Walter and Israel's *General Pathology*. We would reassure the undergraduate that subjects which are contentious or changing rapidly with fashion should not depress him when it comes to answering an examination question. Sensible examiners, and most are, seek evidence that the student has attempted to master the subject which, among other things, requires the reading of textbooks. Sensible examiners soon discern if this has not been done.

Leeds, 1986   P. N. C.
                                                                                          F. G. S.

Acknowledgements

The authors are indebted to Miss Helen Swiercz and Mrs P. M. Docherty for the secretarial work involved in the production of this book. Dr J. Sutton's considerable help with the questions on glomerulonephritis is much appreciated. Mrs D. M. Cowen acted as strict referee for the grammar and comprehensibility of the final production.

Contents

Preface

Questions

Section		
	1. General Pathology	1
	2. Cardiovascular System	4
	3. Respiratory System	6
	4. Haematology	7
	5. Lymphatic System	8
	6. Mouth and Salivary Glands	9
	7. Alimentary System	9
	8. Liver, Gall Bladder and Exocrine Pancreas	12
	9. Nervous System	14
	10. Urinary System	15
	11. Gynaecology	17
	12. Breast	18
	13. Male Reproductive System	19
	14. Endocrine System	20
	15. Skin	22
	16. Bones and Joints	23

Answers

Section		
	1. General Pathology	26
	2. Cardiovascular System	38
	3. Respiratory System	50
	4. Haematology	56
	5. Lymphatic System	62
	6. Mouth and Salivary Glands	67
	7. Alimentary System	69
	8. Liver, Gall Bladder and Exocrine Pancreas	82
	9. Nervous System	88
	10. Urinary System	97
	11. Gynaecology	107
	12. Breast	112
	13. Male Reproductive System	116
	14. Endocrine System	119
	15. Skin	126
	16. Bones and Joints	133

1
Questions

GENERAL PATHOLOGY

1. What is the difference between a genetic and congenital disease?

2. What is the difference between atrophy and involution?

3. What is a fistula?

4. What is an ulcer?

5. What is the difference between hypertrophy and hyperplasia?

6. What is oedema?

7. What are the causes of local and generalised oedema?

8. How is the diagnosis of amyloid disease made?

9. What is amyloidosis and in what conditions does it occur?

10. Does fatty change indicate a specific toxic effect?

11. Which are the commonest cells in which fatty change is seen?

12. What morphological intracellular changes may be seen in a cell undergoing toxic changes?

13. What morphological changes in the nucleus indicate that a cell is dead?

14. What is gangrene?

15. What is a thrombus?

16. What causes thrombosis?

17. How does a wound contract with healing?

18 What are the main stages in the healing of a fracture?

19 What are the chief causes of hypercalcaemia?

20 What is heterotopic calcification?

21 What are the basic defects in scurvy?

22 What are 'collagen diseases'?

23 What determines the sensitivity of a tissue to the damaging effect of ionising irradiation?

24 What is the physiological basis of acute inflammation?

25 What is acute inflammation and by what cardinal signs may it be recognised?

26 What are the pathological differences between acute and chronic suppurative inflammation?

27 What is the relationship between monocytes, histiocytes and macrophages?

28 What is chemotaxis?

29 What are the more important chemical mediators of the inflammatory response?

30 What is the difference between a fibrocyte and a fibroblast?

31 Where are mast cells found? What features make them recognisable and what function do they serve?

32 What skin lesions can be caused by staphylococci? Differentiate them.

33 What structures are infected by *N. gonorrhoeae*?

34 What are the similarities between tetanus and diphtheria?

35 Why is granulation tissue so called?

36 Describe the basic pathological lesion in tuberculosis.

37 Compare the primary with the post-primary (secondary) tuberculous lesion.

38 What parts of the body are commonly affected by *M. tuberculosis* following dissemination from the primary site?

39 Describe the cause and pathology of a gumma.

40 What does the presence of 'sulphur granules' in pus signify and how would you demonstrate them?

41 What are the salient features of gas gangrene?

42 What are the salient features of histoplasmosis?

43 How is histoplasmosis diagnosed?

44 What is an opportunistic infection?

45 What is metaplasia? Give examples.

46 What is the main difference between hyperplasia and neoplasia?

47 What is meant by dysplasia?

48 What is a hamartoma?

49 What is a carcinogen?

50 What is meant by a 'tumour'?

51 What cancers can be caused by ionising radiation in man?

52 What agents are known to be carcinogenic in man and what type of tumour is produced?

53 What is carcinoma *in situ*?

54 What is exfoliative cytology (cytopathology) and what are its clinical applications?

55 How do malignant tumours spread?

56 What is meant by the term 'embryonic tumour'? Where do they occur?

57 What tumours are derived from germ cells?

58 What are the features of teratomata?

59 What are paraneoplastic syndromes?

CARDIOVASCULAR SYSTEM

60 What are the pathological and haemodynamic features of Fallot's Tetrad?

61 What physiological disturbance occurs in children with a patent ductus arteriosus?

62 What is coarctation of the aorta?

63 What is thrombophlebitis?

64 What is the pathology of endarteritis obliterans and in what conditions does it occur?

65 What is atherosclerosis?

66 What factors contribute to the development of atherosclerosis?

67 How does atherosclerosis cause symptomatic disease?

68 Which are the common sites of atherosclerosis?

69 Describe the development of atherosclerosis.

70 What theories have been advanced to explain the development of the atherosclerotic plaque?

71 What is Raynaud's disease?

72 What is Mönckeberg's sclerosis?

73 How does thromboangiitis obliterans (Buerger's disease) differ from atherosclerosis?

74 What are the chief pathological changes in thromboangiitis obliterans?

75 What pathological conditions are associated with degeneration of the media?

76 Why is the aortic arch so commonly affected in tertiary syphilis?

77 What are the causes of aortic incompetence?

78 What are the causes of aortic stenosis?

79 What pathological lesions occur in polyarteritis nodosa?

80 Classify aneurysms according to form.

81 What are the causes of aneurysms?

82 What are valvular vegetations?

83 What are the causes of valvular heart disease?

84 What is the aetiology of rheumatic fever?

85 What part of the heart is affected in acute rheumatic fever?

86 List the organs and tissues affected by acute rheumatic fever.

87 What are the features and complications of chronic rheumatic heart disease?

88 Why is chronic endocarditis a misnomer?

89 What is an Aschoff body?

90 What is the histological appearance of an Aschoff body?

91 Compare acute with subacute bacterial endocarditis.

92 What is infective endocarditis?

93 What are the effects of coronary occlusion?

94 What is angina pectoris?

95 What are the sequelae of a myocardial infarct?

96 How long after a myocardial infarct would you expect to see gross or microscopic changes in the myocardium?

97 What morphological changes in the heart accompany cardiac arrhythmias?

98 What inflammatory conditions may affect the heart?

99 What is meant by the term 'cardiomyopathy'?

100 What are the chief causes and the main clinical and pathological features of heart failure?

101 What conditions cause heart failure?

102 What causes systemic hypertension?

103 What are the pathological results of hypertension?

104 List the causes of pericardial effusion.

105 What is cardiac tamponade?

RESPIRATORY SYSTEM

106 What types of emboli lodge in the pulmonary circulation?

107 Are atelectasis and collapse of the lung the same thing?

108 What are the stages of lobar pneumonia?

109 What are the complications of lobar pneumonia?

110 Compare lobar pneumonia with bronchopneumonia.

111 *Klebsiella* pneumonia has a lobar distribution. How does it differ from the usual lobar pneumonias?

112 What are the salient features of a viral pneumonia?

113 What is the chronic counterpart of non-specific acute bronchitis?

114 What is bronchiectasis and how is it caused?

115 What are the complications of bronchiectasis?

116 Describe the organism which causes *Pneumocystis* pneumonia and the pathogenesis of the condition.

117 What conditions are caused by *Aspergillus fumigatus*?

118 What is an empyema and what can cause it?

119 What may expand the pleural cavity?

120 What are the causes of pleural effusions?

121 How would you classify dust diseases?

122 What are the dangers of inhaling asbestos fibres?

123 What is the difference between emphysema and overinflation of the lung?

124 What varieties of emphysema are recognised?

125 What are the pathognomonic features of chronic bronchitis?

126 What pathologic features are seen in the lungs of a person dying from asthma?

127 What is hyaline membrane disease?

128 What do you understand by the respiratory distress syndrome?

129 What known factors predispose to the development of lung (bronchogenic) cancer?

130 Classify lung cancers.

131 What is the histogenesis of oat-cell carcinoma?

HAEMATOLOGY

132 What is the Arneth count?

133 What conditions are associated with blood eosinophilia?

134 What are the pathologic findings in iron deficiency anaemia?

135 What is the Plummer-Vinson Syndrome?

136 Classify the haemolytic anaemias.

137 What is the relationship between haemolytic anaemias and gall stones?

138 Why might a patient with pernicious anaemia be slightly jaundiced?

139 What are the causes of macrocytic (megaloblastic) anaemia?

140 What pathologic features would be found in a patient dying of a megaloblastic anaemia?

141 What do you understand by bone marrow aplasia?

142 What kinds of leukaemia may occur?

143 What is polycythaemia and what is its cause?

144 What are the pathological features of polycythaemia rubra vera?

145 What is myelosclerosis (myelofibrosis)?

146 What is purpura? What is the difference between a petechial haemorrhage and an ecchymosis?

147 What prevents blood clotting in the circulation?

148 Classify the diseases which cause a haemorrhagic diathesis.

149 What are the causes of hypofibrinogenaemia?

150 What is a schistocyte?

LYMPHATIC SYSTEM

151 What is meant by reactive hyperplasia of a lymph node?

152 What are the causes of lymphatic oedema?

153 What are Warthin-Finkeldey cells?

154 Write a note on the aetiology and pathology of glandular fever.

155 What is Histiocytosis X (or the histiocytoses)?

156 What do you understand by lymphoma?

157 How are non-Hodgkin's lymphomata classified?

158 Describe the Reed-Sternberg cell.

159 How is Hodgkin's lymphoma staged and what is the significance?

160 How is Hodgkin's lymphoma classified?

161 Describe mycosis fungoides.

162 What do splenomegaly and hypersplenism mean?

163 What are the causes of splenomegaly?

164 What lipid storage disorders affect the spleen?

165 What are Gandy-Gamna bodies?

166 Do tumours arise in the thymus?

MOUTH AND SALIVARY GLANDS

167 What is angular cheilitis and what does it signify?

168 What is aphthous ulceration?

169 What are
1. Vincent's angina?
2. Ludwig's angina?

170 What is the pathology of salivary calculi?

171 What is Sjögren's syndrome?

172 What is uveo-parotid fever?

173 What may cause generalised or patchy pigmentation in the mouth?

174 What is meant by the term 'leukoplakia'?

175 Several kinds of neoplasms occur in the salivary glands; describe the commonest one.

ALIMENTARY SYSTEM

176 Which fungi can cause disease in the gastrointestinal tract?

177 What are oesophageal varices?

178 What is reflux oesophagitis?

179 Describe the microscopic changes in peptic oesophagitis.

180 What is a Barrett's ulcer?

181 What is the Mallory-Weiss syndrome?

182 What are the causes of oesophageal obstruction?

183 What types of malignant epithelial tumour occur in the oesophagus?

184 Describe the macroscopic and microscopic appearances of squamous cell tumours of the oesophagus.

185 Which are the most common sites of origin of squamous carcinomata of the oesophagus?

186 Describe the spread of carcinoma of the oesophagus.

187 What types of hiatus hernia are recognised and what are the essential differences between them?

188 What is the difference between a gastric erosion and a gastric ulcer?

189 Describe the microscopic appearance of a chronic peptic ulcer.

190 What are the complications associated with chronic peptic ulceration?

191 What factors appear to influence the frequency of gastric cancer?

192 What are the causes of the Zollinger-Ellison syndrome and what are the chief changes in the gastrointestinal tract?

193 What is meant by the term 'early gastric cancer'?

194 From which common sites do gastric carcinomata arise?

195 What micro-organisms cause acute inflammation of the bowel? Describe the chief pathological changes they produce.

196 How does gastric cancer spread?

197 What pathological changes are associated with giardiasis?

198 What is the effect of a small bowel resection?

199 What is meant by the term 'gluten-induced enteropathy'?

200 What are the chief histological features of gluten-induced enteropathy?

201 What are the chief causes of protein-losing enteropathy?

202 What is the commonest cause of intestinal infarction?

203 What is strangulation of the bowel and what are its causes?

204 What is the commonest cause of ulceration of the small intestine?

205 What are the typical macroscopic appearances in Crohn's disease?

206 What are the typical microscopic changes associated with Crohn's disease?

207 What portion of the gastrointestinal tract is affected in Crohn's disease?

208 What are the pathological features of the Peutz-Jeghers syndrome?

209 What are the chief pathological differences between ulcerative colitis and Crohn's disease?

210 What are the pathological differences between the Peutz-Jeghers syndrome and familial polyposis?

211 What types of malignant tumour arise from the epithelial lining of the small intestine?

212 What is a carcinoid tumour?

213 What are the common complications of acute appendictis?

214 What is meant by the term 'necrotising enterocolitis' and what causes are known?

215 What is Hirschsprung's disease?

216 Define diverticular disease of the colon and explain how it differs from diverticulitis.

217 What aetiological factors are associated with diverticular disease of the colon?

218 What are the chief complications of colonic diverticulosis?

219 What is meant by the term 'back-wash' ileitis?

220 Define a colonic polyp.

221 Classify adenomatous polyps of the large bowel.

222 What conditions of the colon and rectum are quite likely to become malignant?

223 What is the adenoma/carcinoma relationship in the large bowel?

224 Describe the usual macroscopic and microscopic appearances of colorectal cancer.

225 What is meant by Duke's classification of colorectal cancers?

226 What is the relation of carcinoembryonic antigen to carcinoma of the colon?

LIVER & GALL BLADDER

227 What is the Budd-Chiari syndrome?

228 What animal parasites may infest the liver?

229 What is the difference between chronic persistent and chronic active hepatitis?

230 Define and describe cirrhosis of the liver.

231 What patterns of necrosis occur in the liver?

232 Classify the common causes of acquired cirrhosis of the liver.

233 What is primary biliary cirrhosis and what are its pathological features?

234 What is sclerosing cholangitis?

235 What immunologically-associated diseases are liable to occur in a patient with primary biliary cirrhosis?

236 What are the manifestations of hepatocellular failure?

237 What tumours may be found in the liver?

238 What macroscopic and microscopic changes are present in acute cholecystitis?

239 What factors increase the concentration of cholesterol in the bile?

240 What causes gall stone formation?

241 What is the chemical composition of the commoner gall stones?

242 What is meant by the term 'gall stone ileus'?

243 How is acute pancreatitis caused?

244 What are the chief pathological changes in the pancreas in acute pancreatitis?

245 What conditions are commonly associated with acute pancreatitis?

246 Describe the pathological changes associated with chronic pancreatitis.

247 What pathological complications follow a severe attack of pancreatitis?

248 What are the chief features of carcinoma of the pancreas?

NERVOUS SYSTEM

249 What are the pathological complications of a fracture of the skull?

250 What pathological changes occur in brain tissue as a result of a head injury?

251 What is Wallerian degeneration?

252 What metals adversely affect the central nervous system and what is their effect?

253 What is meant by the term 'dysraphic malformation'?

254 What types of spina bifida are recognised?

255 What is the cause of Down's syndrome?

256 What inborn errors of metabolism affect the brain?

257 Name the hereditary neuropathies.

258 What is the difference between Huntington's and Sydenham's chorea?

259 What is the common site of development of subdural haematomata?

260 Where are the common sites in the brain for haemorrhage to occur and what are the predisposing causes?

261 What are the causes of aneurysms of the cerebral arteries?

262 Which artery of the brain is particularly liable to thrombose and what are the consequences?

263 What is marantic thrombosis?

264 What is the gross and microscopic appearance of a cerebral infarct?

265 What is the difference between pachymeningitis and leptomeningitis?

266 What structural changes are associated with

general paralysis of the insane (GPI or chronic syphilitic meningo-encephalitis)?

267 What are the causes of a brain abscess?

268 What are the essential features of cytomegalovirus infection?

269 What is meant by the term 'demyelinating disease'?

270 What are the chief pathological changes in multiple sclerosis?

271 What characteristic histologic feature is found in the brain of patients suffering from Parkinson's disease?

272 Classify the tumours of the nervous system.

273 What is a Schwannoma?

274 What is a meningioma?

URINARY SYSTEM

275 What are the types of polycystic disease of the kidneys?

276 What chemicals are nephrotoxic?

277 What theories have been suggested to account for renal stone formation?

278 What types of stone occur in the upper urinary tract?

279 What factors predispose to the development of renal calculi?

280 What are the pathological complications of renal calculi?

281 How does tuberculosis of the kidney arise?

282 What is meant by the term 'auto-nephrectomy'?

283 What is the commonest cause of acute renal failure?

284 What changes occur in the kidneys in acute tubular necrosis?

285 What is the clinical course of acute tubular necrosis?

286 What is glomerulonephritis?

287 Classify the glomerulonephritides.

288 Why do we trouble to classify the glomerulonephritides?

289 How do the glomerulonephritides usually behave?

290 What are the causes of the glomerulonephritides?

291 How are the immune complexes which occur in the glomerulonephritides detected in the kidney and where are they localised?

292 What is minimal change disease?

293 Describe the glomerulonephritis of Goodpasture's syndrome.

294 What are the renal lesions observed microcopically in malignant hypertension?

295 What structural changes in the kidneys occur in eclampsia?

296 What renal changes are associated with diabetes?

297 What forms of graft rejection affect a transplanted kidney?

298 Describe the changes in the donor kidney associated with chronic rejection of the transplant.

299 Classify the primary tumours of the kidney.

300 Describe the macroscopic and microscopic features of a renal adenocarcinoma.

301 Describe the macroscopic and microscopic appearances of a nephroblastoma.

302 What is hydronephrosis?

303 What is pyelonephritis?

304 What factors predispose to the development of pyelonephritis?

305 Describe the pathology of acute pyelonephritis.

306 What is chronic pyelonephritis?

307 What are the causes of papillary necrosis?

308 What pathological types of cystitis are recognised?

309 What are the common causes of cystitis?

310 What long term changes occur in the bladder as a result of radiation?

311 What are the causes of persistent or recurrent infection of the bladder?

312 Describe Hunner's ulceration.

313 How does *S. haematobium* affect the bladder?

314 What is the histological appearance of schistosomiasis of the bladder?

315 What are the predisposing causes of vesical tumours?

316 What is the gross appearance of a vesical tumour?

317 Describe the microscopic appearance of a vesical tumour.

GYNAECOLOGY

318 What malignant tumours arise in the vagina?

319 Classify endometritis.

320 What is endometriosis and adenomyosis?

321 Describe uterine fibroids.

322 What complications may arise in a uterine fibroid?

323 What do you understand by endometrial hyperplasia?

324 What are the salient clinical and pathological features of carcinoma of the body of the uterus?

325 What is a cervical erosion?

326 What is a cervical polyp?

327 What are the common malignant tumours of the cervix and what is their aetiology?

328 Describe the significance of the histological appearances occurring in the cervix uteri which are considered to herald malignant changes.

329 What are the histological features of cervical epithelial dysplasia (Cervical Intraepithelial Neoplasia; CIN)?

330 What tumours may arise in the ovaries?

331 What is Meig's syndrome?

332 Classify ovarian cysts.

333 What is a Krukenberg tumour?

334 What tumours of placental origin occur?

335 What is a hydatidiform mole?

336 What is an ectopic pregnancy?

BREAST

337 What congenital abnormalities of the breast occur?

338 What may cause a lump in the female breast?

339 What is fibrocystic disease of the breast (mammary dysplasia)?

340 Is mammary dysplasia premalignant?

341 What is the commonest benign breast tumour? Describe it.

342 Do fibroadenomas of breast tend to become malignant?

343 How common is breast carcinoma?

344 What are the aetiological factors involved in the development of breast cancer?

345 Classify breast cancers.

346 What is an inflammatory carcinoma of breast?

347 What is Paget's disease of the nipple?

348 What are oestrogen receptors and what is their significance in breast cancer?

349 Can a man develop carcinoma of the breast?

350 What are the likely reasons for swellings in the male breast?

351 What are the causes and appearances of gynaecomastia?

MALE REPRODUCTIVE

352 What are the common causal organisms of acute prostatitis?

353 What types of granulomatous prostatitis have been described?

354 Which group of prostatic glands is affected in benign hyperplasia?

355 Describe the microscopic appearance of nodular hyperplasia of the prostate.

356 What are the chief pathological complications associated with benign prostatic hyperplasia?

357 Where in the prostate does carcinoma develop?

358 What are the modes of spread of prostatic cancer?

359 Classify the causes of orchitis.

360 What types of non-germinal tumours of the testes occur?

361 What are the common germ-cell tumours of the testes?

362 What is a yolk-sac tumour?

363 Do lymphomata occur in the testes?

364 What type of testicular tumour is associated with the appearance of 'tumour markers'?

365 Describe a hard chancre of the penis.

366 What conditions may precede the development of carcinoma of the penis?

367 What is Fournier's gangrene?

368 What was the first occupational cancer described?

ENDOCRINE SYSTEM

369 What is a craniopharyngioma?

370 What is the pathological basis of Sheehan's syndrome?

371 What percentage of intracranial tumours arise from the adenohypophysis and what are their respective cells of origin?

372 How do tumours of the adenohypophysis produce clinical effects?

373 What is the pathological basis of diabetes insipidus?

374 What is acromegaly?

375 What types of goitre are recognised?

376 What is meant by the term 'multinodular goitre'?

377 What is meant by the term 'simple or colloid goitre'?

378 What are the causes of a colloid goitre?

379 Describe the aetiology of primary thyrotoxicosis.

380 What are the histological appearances of a toxic goitre?

381 What is meant by the term 'toxic adenoma'?

382 What are the pathological varieties of auto-immune thyroiditis?

383 Describe the gross and microscopic appearances in lymphadenoid goitre (Hashimoto's disease).

384 What is Riedel's thyroiditis?

385 Classify tumours of the thyroid.

386 What are the chief pathological features of follicular carcinoma of the thyroid?

387 What are the chief pathological features of a papillary carcinoma of the thyroid?

388 Describe the chief features of medullary carcinoma of the thyroid.

389 What conditions lead to the development of secondary hyperparathyroidism?

390 What are the types of hyperparathyroidism?

391 What pathological changes occur in hyperparathyroidism?

392 What types of tumours originate from the pancreatic islet cells?

393 Describe the Zollinger-Ellison syndrome.

394 What causes acute destruction of the adrenal gland?

395 What are the causes of chronic destruction of the adrenal glands?

396 What is Addison's disease?

397 Describe the non-chromaffin tumours of the adrenal medulla.

398 What is a phaeochromocytoma?

399 What syndromes are associated with the excessive secretion of cortical adrenal hormones?

400 What is the essential pathological difference between Cushing's syndrome and Cushing's disease?

401 What is primary hyperaldosteronism (Conn's syndrome)?

402 What are the multiple endocrine neoplasia (MEN) syndromes?

SKIN

403 What is the difference between a furuncle and a carbuncle?

404 What are the differences between impetigo and erysipelas?

405 What is dermatitis?

406 What are the chief pathological differences between acute and chronic dermatitis?

407 What pathological lesion is caused by the pox and herpes virus?

408 Do circulating antibodies develop in the pemphigoid group of disorders?

409 What is meant by the term 'fish-skin disease'?

410 What are the characteristic pathological features of psoriasis?

411 What are sebaceous, epidermoid and dermoid cysts?

412 What are the chief pathological features of acne vulgaris?

413 What tumours can arise in the epidermis?

414 What is a wart?

415 Compare condylomata lata and condylomata acuminata.

416 What is a keratoacanthoma?

417 What is molluscum contagiosum?

418 What is a fibrous histiocytoma?

419 Describe a rodent ulcer.

420 Describe a typical squamous carcinoma of the skin.

421 What lesions of melanocytes occur in the skin?

422 What histological types of malignant naevus cell tumours occur and what is their significance?

BONES & JOINTS

423 What are the bacteria which most frequently infect bone?

424 Describe the evolution of osteomyelitis of staphylococcal origin.

425 What micro-organisms other than the *Staphylococcus aureus* can cause acute osteomyelitis?

426 What is Pott's disease of the spine?

427 What pathological change is associated with avitaminosis C in the adult?

428 What are the chief causes of Vitamin D deficiency?

429 What is rickets?

430 What bones are particularly affected in rickets?

431 What are the chief histopathological features of rickets?

432 What is the chief histopathological change in the skeleton in osteomalacia?

433 What biochemical changes occur in osteomalacia?

434 What are the chief clinical effects of osteomalacia?

435 What is osteosclerosis and what are its causes?

436 Define osteoporosis.

437 What are the causes of osteoporosis?

438 What are the chief histological changes in osteoporosis?

439 What is the clinical importance of osteoporosis?

440 What is renal osteodystrophy?

441 What is meant by the term 'osteochondrosis' (osteochondritis juvenilis or avascular necrosis of bone)?

442 What is osteitis fibrosa cystica?

443 What biochemical changes are found in Paget's disease of bone?

444 What are the main histological features of Paget's disease of bone?

445 What are the commonest malignant tumours occurring in bone?

446 Classify the commoner primary tumours which arise in bone.

447 Describe the gross and microscopic appearance of an osteogenic sarcoma.

448 What are the main features of a giant cell tumour of bone (osteoclastoma)?

449 What is a Ewing's tumour?

450 Describe cartilage tumours.

451 What is a chordoma?

452 Describe the pathological development of suppurative arthritis.

453 What organisms are commonly responsible for suppurative arthritis?

454 What pathological changes occur in the joints in rheumatoid arthritis?

455 Describe the features of rheumatoid arthritis which suggest that it is due to an immunological cause.

456 What diseases may be associated with a rheumatoid type of arthritis?

457 What is Still's disease?

458 What is osteoarthrosis?

459 What factors contribute to the development of osteoarthrosis?

460 What metabolic conditions cause arthritis?

461 Describe the changes associated with haemophilic arthritis.

462 What is a neuropathic (Charcot's) joint?

2
Answers

GENERAL PATHOLOGY

1 A genetic disease is a condition which is determined by Mendelian factors. It may present after birth e.g. mucoviscidosis. A congenital disease is present at birth whatever the cause and may be genetic but not necessarily so. Thalidomide and maternal rubella during pregnancy cause congenital but not genetic defects.

2 Atrophy is usually considered to be pathological although it may be argued whether the atrophic changes of old age constitute a pathological state. Involution is physiological and is exemplified by branchial cleft disappearance during embryogenesis and the uterus reverting to normal size *post-partum*.

3 A fistula is an abnormal communication between the lumena of two hollow viscera or between the lumen of a viscus and the exterior. Examples are the vesico-colic fistula complicating colonic diverticulitis and fistula-in-ano.

4 An ulcer is a break in the continuity of an epithelial or endothelial surface.

5 In both cases, the organ or tissue is enlarged due, in the case of hypertrophy, to an increase in size of the constituent cells and, in hyperplasia, to an increase in the number of cells.

6 Oedema is the accumulation of excessive fluid in the interstitial tissues although in the case of pulmonary oedema the fluid is in alveolar spaces. Generalised oedema is frequently associated with pleural, pericardial and peritoneal effusions.

7 1. Local oedema:
a. pulmonary due to
   (i) left sided heart failure
   (ii) cerebral damage

    (iii) irritants; gases, gastric contents etc.
    (iv) infections, particularly viral
    (v) oxygen toxicity
b. acute inflammation
c. hypersensitivity reactions
d. obstruction of venous return
e. obstruction of lymphatic drainage

2. Generalised oedema:
a. congestive heart failure
b. renal failure
c. starvation
d. liver failure
e. adrenal hormones causing salt retention i.e. Cushing's syndrome
f. hypothyroidism
g. pregnancy

8 By biopsy of the gums or rectal mucosa. Amyloid stains with Congo Red and produces an apple green colour in polarised light.

9 Amyloidosis is a condition in which one of several varieties of abnormal glycoprotein is deposited in the tissues. It is most commonly an idiopathic condition but it may be secondary to:
  1. rheumatoid arthritis
  2. myelomatosis
  3. chronic sepsis e.g. chronic osteomyelitis or bronchiectasis
Death from amyloidosis frequently occurs as a result of renal or cardiac failure caused by its deposition in these organs.

10 No. Fatty changes may occur following almost any kind of toxic insult including anoxia.

11 Hepatocytes, myocardial fibres and renal tubular epithelial cells.

12 Fatty change, cloudy swelling, vascular and hyaline degeneration, all of which are reversible. However, in some conditions such as Niemann-Pick disease the cells irreversibly store large amounts of abnormal substances such as sphingomyelin.

13 1. Pyknosis
    2. Karyorrhexis
    3. Karyolysis

14 Pathologically, gangrene is necrosis of an organ with superadded putrefaction. Clinically, there are two types. In dry gangrene the organ, usually a limb, becomes mummified in the absence of infection. In wet gangrene, necrosis and putrefaction occur due to superadded infection.

15 The formation in the circulating blood of a solid mass composed of the constituents of the blood, chiefly fibrin and platelets with an admixture of erythrocytes and leucocytes.

16 1. Damage to, or destruction of endothelium or endocardium.
    2. Changes in blood flow caused by:
       a. slowing of the blood stream
       b. eddy currents
       c. increase in blood viscosity
    3. Alterations in the constituents of the blood:
       a. thrombocytosis
       b. increase in clotting factors
       c. hyperlipidaemia

17 Not, as was previously thought, due to the contraction of collagen laid down by the fibroblasts but due to the removal of oedema and contraction of granulation tissue before it develops into a collagenous scar. Fibroblasts or myofibroblasts in the granulation tissue are responsible for its contraction.

18 1. Haematoma forms at the broken ends of the bone.
    2. Acute inflammation occurs.
    3. The granulocytes and histiocytes remove the debris, i.e. the haematoma and any necrotic tissue including fragments of bone.
    4. Granulation tissue forms between and around the bone ends after removal of the debris.
    5. Cartilage and bone are laid down in this granulation tissue which becomes hard and is consequently called callus. The cartilage ossifies and the bone laid down is known as woven bone because of the lack of normal lamellar organisation. It occupies both the original marrow cavity as well as bridging the compact bone ends.
    6. The woven bone is resorbed and replaced by lamellar bone.
    7. During 6., remodelling occurs simultaneously

so that, in a properly reduced fracture, no deformity remains.

19
1. Osteolytic malignant disease.
2. Primary, secondary or tertiary hyperparathyroidism.
3. Vitamin D intoxication.
4. Milk-alkali syndrome.

20 Heterotopic calcification is the deposition of calcium salts in tissues other than osteoid or teeth. There are two types:
1. dystrophic calcification when calcification occurs in dead or dying tissue
2. metastatic calcification in which calcification occurs in normal tissue due to hypercalcaemia from any cause

21 Scurvy is caused by vitamin C deficiency. A deficient intake results in a failure of collagen synthesis by the fibroblasts and an increase in the amount of degraded polymerised mucopolysaccharide in the connective tissue.

22 The collagen or connective tissue diseases are:
1. acute rheumatic fever
2. rheumatoid arthritis
3. systemic lupus erythematosus
4. polyarteritis nodosa
5. scleroderma

These conditions were once considered to be autoimmune diseases during the course of which collagen underwent fibrinoid necrosis. This term is a misnomer since collagen, being inanimate, cannot undergo necrosis. No evidence, however, exists to show that auto-antibodies to collagen form and a common pathogenesis for these diseases is now in doubt. Many consider that they represent an immune-complex type of allergy, degeneration of collagen being a secondary phenomenon.

23 The chief factor is the proportion of cells in a tissue undergoing mitosis since cells are sensitive to ionising irradiation during this part of the cell cycle. Particularly sensitive tissues are, therefore, those in which frequent mitoses are occurring, e.g. the germinal cells of the ovaries and testes, the haemopoietic system and the intestinal epithelial cells.

24 The triple response of Lewis. Vasodilatation of the capillaries and arterioles is the keynote. This permits the exudation of fluid containing chemical mediators and, later, the migration of inflammatory cells, mainly granulocytes, into the tissues.

25 Acute inflammation is a defence mechanism of the body to a variety of injuries, including trauma, toxic substances and infections. The cardinal signs were described by Celsus, a Roman living in Provence in the 1st century AD, as rubor, calor, dolor and tumor, in other words inflammation is a red, hot, painful, swelling. At a later date it was recognised that loss of function was also associated with acute inflammation.

26 Acute inflammation is of short duration and destruction of tissue is minimal, permitting resolution; a virtual return to normal. The inflammatory cell involved is predominantly the neutrophil granulocyte. In chronic inflammation, more tissue is destroyed and mononuclear cells; lymphocytes, plasmacytes and histiocytes, also take part. The destroyed tissue is replaced by granulation tissue and healing is by fibrosis leaving a scar.

27 They are cells of the reticulo-endothelial system, recently re-named the mononuclear phagocyte system, and are generally considered to have a common origin and to be interconvertible. The precursor cell is in the bone marrow. This produces the promonocyte which, in turn, produces the monocyte which enters the bloodstream. Monocytes may then migrate into the connective tissues when they are called histiocytes, meaning 'tissue cells'. Showing phagocytic properties, they may also be called macrophages. The Kupffer cells in the liver, the alveolar macrophages in the lung, the macrophages lining the sinusoids of the spleen and lymph nodes and possibly the microglial cells all belong to the mononuclear phagocyte system.

28 It is the directional movement of a cell in response to a chemical substance and, in the context of acute inflammation, it is applied to the neutrophil granulocytes and histiocytes.

29 1. Amines; histamine and 5-HT.

2. Kinins.
3. Kinin precursors (enzymes); kallikrein and plasmin.
4. Certain products of the complement system.
5. Certain components of polymorphs.
6. Prostaglandins.

30 A fibrocyte is a mesenchymal cell, elongated in shape with a thin nucleus, which is quiescent. A fibroblast is its active counterpart, larger in size, which produces collagen.

31 Mast cells are found in the collagenous connective tissues anywhere in the body. They are recognised by their intracytoplasmic granules which stain metachromatically with stains such as toluidine blue and Giemsa. The granules consist of heparin and histamine and the cells, therefore, are important in inflammatory and anaphylactic responses.

32 1. Impetigo, presents as superficial pustules in the epidermis.
2. Folliculitis, when the superficial part of a hair follicle is infected.
3. Furuncles, when the whole shaft and root of the hair follicle is infected and an abscess forms.
4. A localised suppurative abcess may occur in the dermis.
5. Carbuncles, when an ill-defined, subcutaneous, suppurative process occurs usually producing several confluent abcesses with multiple discharging sinuses.

33 In the male, the urethra, prostate, seminal vesicles and epididymis. In the female in whom the infection is less severe, the urethra, cervix, uterine tubes and pelvic peritoneum.

In prepubertal girls vaginitis may occur due to the neutral pH of the vagina. In the mature woman, due to oestrogen secretion, the pH is normally acidic and thus antibacterial.

34 Both organisms proliferate locally and cause symptoms by the liberation of their exotoxins.

35 Granulation tissue is so called from its appearance on the skin surface where lost epidermis and dermis is replaced by capillaries bathed in serum

and pus. Capillary loops grow outwards in the direction of the skin surface and are seen as red granules among the pus when looking down on the ulcerated area.

36 Neutrophils first appear at the site of infection and are soon replaced by macrophages and lymphocytes. As the lesion develops the following zones from centre to periphery become recognisable and constitute a tubercle:
  1. a central zone of caseous necrosis in which organisms may be found
  2. a zone composed of macrophages which, having a supposed similarity to the cells of the stratum spinosum of the skin are called epithelioid cells, scattered among which are the multinucleate giant cells, the Langhans' cells. Tubercle bacilli are most likely to be seen in this zone
  3. a zone of lymphocytes beyond which may be found granulation or fibrous tissue depending on the age of the lesion, the amount of tissue loss and the stage of healing

37 Primary and secondary tuberculosis occur at the same sites, most frequently the lung or small intestine, but whereas a primary lesion tends to heal spontaneously, a post-primary lesion, in the absence of treatment, tends to progress to produce cavitation in the affected tissues.

  Both, however, if progressive, spread in a similar fashion but primary lesions tend to be associated with a greater degree of enlargement of the nodes draining the site than in the case of secondary lesions. Miliary tuberculosis, the result of blood-stream dissemination of the bacilli in a susceptible individual, is more common in primary than secondary tuberculosis.

38 From the primary site of infection, lung, intestine or rarely skin, bacilli may spread to the adjacent lymph nodes via the lymphatics and then by the blood stream to the brain, meninges, the genito-urinary tract, bones and joints. When the primary focus is the lung, sputum when swallowed may infect the bowel or when expectorated may affect the trachea, vocal cords or tongue.

39 A gumma is typically the lesion of tertiary syphilis. It is an area of coagulative necrosis which

can occur in almost any organ and eventually becomes fibrosed and rubbery hard (*gummi* in German = rubber). The lesion is an area of ischaemic infarction due to hypersensitivitiy to the spirochaete and although the necrosis is similar to caseation, the tissue is mummified and its original architecture is still descernible. Numerous inflammatory cells, lymphocytes, plasma cells, histiocytes and occasional giant cells are seen. Fibroblasts then lay down collagen. Common sites are liver, testis, subcutaneous tissues and bone.

40 'Sulphur granules' are colonies of actinomyces. They are demonstrated by shaking a drop of pus in a test-tube of water. The colonies are then seen suspended as tiny yellow-green flakes similar to powdered sulphur grains.

41 It is caused by mixed infection with various proteolytic and saccharolytic clostridia which produce powerful necrotising exotoxins. Although clostridia are ubiquitous, this condition is rare in civilian life because wounds have to be heavily contaminated by dirt or devitalised tissue for the organisms to proliferate. Contamination is from spores in soil or faeces, the organisms becoming vegetative in anaerobic conditions. During infection, gas is produced and crepitation can be felt in subcutaneous tissue and muscle. Local effects include gangrene of tissues and limbs and systemically there is severe toxaemia.

42 Histoplasmosis, which occurs mainly in children, is caused by a saprophytic fungus, *Histoplasma capsulatum* or *duboisi* which grows as a mycelium in the soil and as a yeast at 37°. Infection probably occurs by inhalation, the lungs being affected first, after which there may be haematological spread to the spleen, lymph nodes, liver and bone marrow. The basic lesion is one of necrosis with no evidence of caseation, the yeast being found surrounded by macrophages. The disease is not transmitted from man to man.

43 1. By examination of the sputum, blood or bone marrow, in all of which the yeast-like organism may be seen.
    2. Serologically
        a. complement-fixing antibodies develop in the serum.

b. the histoplasmin test, a skin test, when positive indicates not only current but also previous infection.

44 In immunodeficient individuals infection by saprophytic or commensal organisms may cause severe disease. Many pulmonary infections of this type are caused by fungi e.g. *Aspergillus fumigatus* and *Candida albicans*. Immunodeficiency may be a product of diseases such as leukaemia, lymphomata and AIDS or induced by drugs as the glucocorticoids or cytotoxic agents.

45 Metaplasia is a change from one type of differentiated tissue to another.
Examples are:
1. the respiratory epithelium which is normally composed of pseudostratified columnar epithelium may change to a squamous epithelium as a result of smoking or the inhalation of dust or into an epithelium predominantly composed of goblet cells in chronic bronchitis
2. the transitional epithelium lining the urinary tract may change to stratified squamous in the presence of stones
3. the glandular epithelium of the gall bladder may become squamous when calculi are present
4. metaplasia can occur in connective tissues e.g. osseous or cartilaginous metaplasia in fibrous tissue

46 Hyperplasia is a limited overgrowth of a tissue as a result of the excessive action of a specific stimulus. It may be considered physiological. Neoplasia is an excess growth of cells in a tissue, commonly for no known reason, which may stop after a time in the case of benign neoplasms or continue unabated at the primary and secondary sites in the case of malignant neoplasms.

47 Strictly this term should be applied to a disordered growth in a tissue or organ, e.g. mammary dysplasia, broncho-pulmonary dysplasia, renal dysplasia, fibrous dysplasia of bone and, at the microscopic level, dysplastic colonic glands. However, the term is also applied to individual cells having an atypical or bizarre appearance. Since this may represent a preneoplastic change, or even neoplasia, the word 'dysplasia' has come

to have a distinct premalignant connotation which is not necessarily true.

48 A hamartoma is a disorderly but limited overgrowth in an organ or tissue of well-differentiated cells which are normally present in that organ.

49 Any agent, physical, chemical or parasitic which causes a malignant growth to develop. Many carcinogens are species-specific, and reference to them should refer to the animal.

50 Originally a tumour meant any lump, inflammatory, neoplastic or otherwise. Nowadays it is synonymous with 'neoplasm' or 'new growth'. The commonly accepted definition of a neoplasm is that of Willis who stated that a tumour is an abnormal mass of tissue the growth of which exceeds and is uncoordinated with that of the normal tissues and which persists in the same excessive manner after the cessation of the stimuli which evoked the change. However, on rare occasions, malignant neoplasms have been known to regress spontaneously.

51 1. Squamous carcinoma of the skin.
    2. Osteogenic sarcoma of bone.
    3. The leukaemias.
    4. Bronchogenic carcinoma.
    5. Thyroid carcinoma.

52 1. Polycyclic hydrocarbons found in tar or shale oil; skin cancer and, from tobacco smoke; bronchial cancer.
    2. Some aniline dyes used in the dyestuffs and rubber industries; urothelial tumours.
    3. Crocidolite, one of the three varieties of asbestos; mesotheliomata of the pleura or peritoneum.
    4. Wood dust when inhaled; adenocarcinoma of the nasal mucosa or paranasal sinuses.
    5. Vinyl chloride, in the plastic industry; angiosarcoma of the liver.
    6. Ionising irradiation; neoplastic changes in various sites.
    7. Arsenic; skin cancer.
    8. Ultraviolet light in fair skinned individuals may cause squamous or basal cell carcinoma and melanoma.
    9. Infections,

    a. viral cancer is well-recognised in animals, in man the association is less clear but examples in which viruses are important in man include:
      (i) Burkitt's lymphoma;
      (ii) nasopharyngeal cancer;
      (iii) Kaposi's sarcoma.
    b. metazoan parasites such as *Schistosoma haematobium*, causing cancer of the bladder.

53 A neoplasm of epithelial origin, the cells of which are morphologically malignant but which have not breached the basement membrane. An example is intra-epithelial cancer of the skin, Bowen's disease.

54 Exfoliative cytology is the study of cells shed from epithelial or mesothelial surfaces or cells obtained by fine needle aspiration of solid tumours. The purpose, nearly always, is to detect or exclude the presence of a malignant neoplasm. This diagnostic tool was developed originally for the investigation of the cervix uteri.

    However, sputum and urine specimens are commonly examined in order to exclude or confirm the presence of bronchial or urothelial cancers. Examination of pleural, pericardial or ascitic fluid may also reveal the presence of the malignant cells which cause these effusions.

55 1. By direct invasion of adjacent structures, including perineural spread.
    2. By lymphatic vessels.
    3. By blood vessels.
    4. Across body cavities; pleural, peritoneal, the ventricular system of the brain and the subarachnoid space.
    5. Rarely, through cells—tumour cells are sometimes seen insinuating themselves along skeletal muscle fibres.

56 'Embryonic tumours' occur in infancy and childhood. They occur in:
    1. the kidney, the nephroblastoma or Wilm's tumour
    2. the adrenal or sympathetic ganglia, the neuroblastoma

3. the cerebellum and 4th ventricle, the medulloblastoma
4. the retina, the retinoblastoma
5. the liver, the hepatoblastoma, very rare
6. the lung, pulmonary blastoma, very rare

57 These tumours commonly arise in the gonads and rarely in sites occupied by the gonads during their development. They are:
1. Seminoma in testis and dysgerminoma in ovary.
2. Tetratoma.
3. Choriocarcinoma (extra-uterine).
4. Yolk sac tumour (endodermal sinus tumour when in ovary and orchioblastoma in testis).

58 Teratomata consist of multiple tissues foreign to the part from which they arise. Most occur in the gonads which led to the concept that they were monsters which developed parthenogenetically from an ovum or sperm but they can also arise in the mediastinum and sacrum.

Such tumours may contain well-differentiated epithelial, mesothelial and endothelial elements producing such structures as hair, teeth and gastrointestinal glands

If only epithelial structures are involved the tumours are cystic and classified as dermoids.

Whereas many teratomata of the ovary are cystic and benign, testicular teratomata are more usually solid, poorly-differentiated and malignant.

59 They are a variety of unrelated systemic conditions occurring in patients suffering from malignant disease, commonly due to the excretion of hormones not usually associated with the tissue of tumour origin e.g. an oat-cell cancer of the bronchus. This tumour may secret 5-HT producing the carcinoid syndrome, ACTH producing Cushing's syndrome, a melanocyte-stimulating hormone, or an antidiuretic hormone. The secretion of 5-HT is, however, not entirely inappropriate since the cell of origin is the Feyrter cell. Paraneoplastic syndromes not caused by hormone secretion include neuropathies, encephalopathies, myopathies and thrombotic conditions.

CARDIOVASCULAR SYSTEM

60
1. Stenosis of the pulmonary valve (or infundibular part of right ventricle).
2. Right ventricular hypertrophy due to increased pressure in that chamber, resulting from 1.
3. A high interventricular defect just below the aortic and pulmonary valves.
4. Over-riding of the aorta to the right (dextroposition) so that the reduced blood from the right ventricle, which cannot be ejected through the stenosed pulmonary valve, passes through the defect (3) to mix with left ventricular blood and thence through the aortic valve to the aorta.

A variable degree of cyanosis occurs, depending on the severity of the above abnormalities.

61 The patent ductus is usually narrow, a little blood flows from the aorta to the pulmonary artery and there are no symptoms at first. With time, in severe cases, right sided heart failure occurs.

In some cases there is pulmonary hypertension and the blood flow is from pulmonary artery to aorta. The ductus enters the aorta just distal to the left subclavian artery so reduced blood reaches the lower but not upper extremities. In this case the result is cyanosed nail beds of the toes but not the fingers.

Finally, subacute bacterial endocarditis may affect a patent ductus arteriosus.

62 Coarctation of the aorta is congenital and usually occurs just distal to the origin of the left subclavian artery. This condition is associated with normal pulses in the upper limbs and reduced pulses in the lower. The condition may present as an acute emergency in childhood or go unnoticed until found incidentally in adult life.

63 Thrombophlebitis is caused by injury or infection of a vein. Infection may occur in the veins of the diploë and dura during the course of suppurative otitis media, in the uterine veins in puerperal sepsis and in the veins of the bone marrow in osteomyelitis. In aseptic thrombophlebitis the thrombus within the affected vein becomes organised and later recanalised. In infective thrombophlebitis infected thrombi may fragment producing a pyaemia.

64 Endarteritis obliterans consists of the narrowing of arterial or arteriolar lumena by concentric subintimal laminae of cellular connective tissue which finally obliterate them. It occurs normally at birth in the umbilical arteries, in the ductus arteriosus and in the involuting post-partum uterus. It occurs pathologically in vessels in the base of chronic peptic ulcers, in the walls of tuberculous cavities, in syphilis and as a result of irradiation.

65 Atherosclerosis is defined by the World Health Organisation as a condition in which variable changes develop in the internal layers of arteries. These changes, which originate in the intima and extend into the media, consist of focal accumulations of lipids, complex carbohydrates, blood and blood products, fibrous tissue and calcium salts.

66
1. Age; progressive symptomatic disease is only common after 40 years of age.
2. Sex; in females atherosclerosis rarely occurs in the premenopausal period.
3. Environment; the mortality from this disease is much lower in the Third World than in the highly industrialised Western World.
4. A high serum cholesterol, such as occurs in diabetes, myxoedema, the nephrotic syndrome and familial xanthosis.
5. Hypertension.
6. Smoking.

67 Atherosclerosis causes symptomatic disease by depriving tissues or organs of blood. The effects of gradual occlusion differ according to the tissue or organ affected, e.g. involvement of the cerebral arteries causes cerebral atrophy followed by dementia; of the renal arteries, renal scarring causing hypertension; of the coronary arteries, myocardial fibrosis associated with angina; of the lower limb arteries, ischaemia of the muscles and skin causing claudication and finally gangrene.

68 Atherosclerosis can occur at almost any part of an artery but it is commoner around the ostia of arterial branches and in small vessels which are not well supported externally.

69 Stage I, a fatty streak composed of smooth muscle

cells containing fat develops immediately beneath the intima.

Stage II, confluent smooth yellowish plaques several millimetres in diameter, which are composed of lipid, can be seen. At the periphery of such a plaque the lipid is intracellular but in the centre it forms a structureless extracellular amorphous mass. The plaque is separated from the endothelium by a layer of hyaline fibres.

Stage III. Around and in between the plaques widespread proliferation of fibrous tissue occurs causing irregular thickening of the intima. In advanced disease the endothelium disappears leaving the underlying lipid exposed, producing the atheromatous ulcer upon which mural thrombosis may develop. Calcification, particularly in plaques in the distal aorta, occurs at this stage. Degeneration of the media leads to aneurysmal dilatation of the affected vessel.

70 1. The thrombogenic theory. This postulates that repeated episodic mural thrombi occur, each of which, by being covered by endothelium, are incorporated into the intima where they cause fibrosis and accumulate lipid.
    2. The filtration theory. This, the more universally accepted theory, postulates that lipid is filtered from the blood into the intimal and subintimal zones.

71 Raynaud's disease is a vasospastic phenomenon of unknown aetiology affecting the fingers. However, similar vascular phenomena followed by structural changes in the digital arteries occur in a variety of occupations, e.g. in those using vibrating tools and in patients with scleroderma or poisoned by ergot. In these secondary conditions fibrous thickening of the intima of the digital arteries occurs together with thrombosis leading to severe trophic changes and eventually gangrene.

72 A degenerative disease of the large arteries mainly, but not always, occurring in the elderly and associated with dystrophic calcification of the media, the intima remaining normal. The vessel becomes rigid without any reduction in the size of the lumen.

73 1. It occurs at a lower age group, affecting males between 25–40 years of age.

2. Larger vessels are unaffected.
3. In both the upper and lower limbs the digital vessels may be affected.
4. Superficial phlebitis may precede the arterial changes.
5. Lipid is not present in significant amounts in the walls of affected arteries.

Despite these differences some authorities believe that Buerger's disease is simply atherosclerosis in the young.

74 The affected vessels are not dilated but are firm to the touch and frequently adherent to the adjacent venae comitantes. The microscopic appearance depends upon the stage of the disease. In the early stages polymorphonuclear leucocytes infiltrate the whole thickness of wall of an affected vessel. Later, thrombosis occurs and occludes the lumen. The thrombus is then organised, the fibrous tissue extending outwards to involve adjacent structures including the veins. Recanalisation does occur but the blood supply to the tissues distal to an affected segment is chiefly dependent upon collaterals.

75 1. Erdheim's medial degeneration.
2. Marfan's syndrome.

In both, degeneration and cystic changes occur in the media. The elastic tissue and muscle are replaced by a mucoid substance. In both, the vascular abnormality only becomes apparent when an intimal tear immediately above the aortic cusps leads to the development of a dissecting aneurysm.

Erdheim's is a condition of unknown aetiology. Marfan's syndrome is inherited through a dominant autosomal gene and is also associated with the defective formation of collagen and elastic tissue throughout the body causing, in addition to the vascular abnormality, laxity of various ligaments.

76 Because of the rich lymphatic supply to this part of the aorta. The lymphatics provide a pathway for the treponemes from the mediastinal lymph nodes to the vessel wall. The basic lesion is an arteritis of the vasa vasorum ramifying in the adventitia.

77 1. Rheumatic heart disease in which the aortic

cusps become thickened and contracted.
2. Atherosclerosis.
3. Marfan's syndrome.
4. Syphilitic aortitis which specifically affects the ascending part of the aorta.

78 Aortic stenosis may be congenital or acquired.
1. Congenital aortic stenosis is most commonly due to the replacement of the three valve cusps by a single diaphragm-like membrane with a central foramen. Less commonly it is due to a subvalvular membrane.
2. Acquired aortic stenosis is most commonly seen in chronic rheumatic heart disease when organisation of the vegetations formed in the acute stage produce adhesions between cusps and deformity of the valve. Less commonly it results from the fibrosis and subsequent calcification of congenitally bicuspid valves.

79 The earliest lesions consist of foci of fibrinoid necrosis in the intima and media of the small and medium sized arteries accompanied by a polymorphonuclear infiltration of the whole thickness of the vessel wall. Superadded thrombosis or haemorrhage may occur in the acute phase. In the chronic phase the necrotic vessel wall is replaced by fibrous tissue infiltrated with lymphocytes, plasma cells and macrophages and the thrombus becomes organised. Polyarteritis nodosa chiefly affects the vessels of the kidneys, gut, heart, liver, pancreas and nervous system. When the heart and kidneys are affected death may occur rapidly but the disease can also run an episodic course.

80 1. Fusiform, when the entire circumference of the artery dilates.
2. Saccular, when only one part of the circumference is distended.
3. False, caused by injury to the vessel wall. The aneurysmal sac is formed of granulation tissue developing in the haematoma surrounding the injured vessel. An arterio-venous aneurysm may result when such a fistula occurs.
4. Racemose, aneurysmal dilatation arising from a communication between arteries and veins, commonly seen on the scalp as a cirsoid aneurysm. This may be the result of trauma.
5. Dissecting, when the media degenerates and blood tracks through an intimal tear into it.

The bulge in the vessel is thus caused by blood or blood clot.

81 1. Congenital. Strictly, congenital aneurysms do not occur but the term has gained general acceptance to describe those aneurysms which arise on the circle of Willis and its branches. Such an aneurysm is not present at birth but develops later because of a congenital deficiency of the smooth muscle of the media.
2. Acquired:
   a. degenerative —atherosclerosis
                   —Erdheim's medial degeneration
                   —Marfan's syndrome
   b. infective   —mycotic
                   —syphilitic
   c. traumatic   —surgery to a major artery may lead to the development of a false aneurysm, an aneurysmal varix or varicose aneurysm
   d. cirsoid   —this variety occurs on the scalp and may be congenital but is usually traumatic. While considered congenital, it may be the result of a birth injury

82 Valvular vegetations are formed by deposits of platelets and fibrin on the cusps of the valves of the heart. They occur more commonly in the left side of the heart than the right and affect the mitral more frequently than the aortic valve. In acute rheumatic endocarditis the vegetations are small excrescences in the line of apposition of the affected cusps, hence it is believed that trauma leading to ulceration of the endocardium precedes the development of the vegetations. In acute and subacute bacterial endocarditis, the vegetations also contain micro-organisms.

83 1. Rheumatic heart disease in the acute or chronic stage. In the acute stage vegetations develop on the valve cusps and in the chronic stage scarring and deformity of the affected valves occur.
2. Acute infective endocarditis.
3. Subacute bacterial endocarditis, an infection of

deformed valves by organisms of normally low pathogenicity.
4. Atheroma of the mitral valve associated with fibrosis and calcification.
5. Libman-Sacks endocarditis occurring in patients with systemic lupus erythematosus.
6. Calcification of the aortic valve not associated with atherosclerosis.
7. Fibrosis of the tricuspid and pulmonary valves in association with the carcinoid syndrome.
8. Marantic endocarditis occurring in terminally ill patients.

84 Rheumatic fever is caused by *Streptococcus haemolyticus*, Lancefield Group A. It is believed that antibodies stimulated by the exotoxin of this bacterium act as auto-antibodies against the patient's own myocardial fibres. This hypothesis is supported by:
1. the time lapse of 2–4 weeks between the onset of the streptococcal throat infection and rheumatic fever
2. patients developing rheumatic fever have a higher titre of streptococcal antibodies than those who do not
3. streptococcal antigens can be found in the myocardial fibres.

This hypothesis cannot explain all aspects of the disease since collagen, particularly of the endocardium and periarticular tissues is also affected.

The disease is commoner in children living in poorer social conditions.

85 Rheumatic fever causes a pancarditis; the pericardium, myocardium and endocardium being involved.

86 1. In the heart, the endocardium, myocardium and pericardium.
2. The joints and tendon sheaths.
3. The subcutaneous tissues.
4. The skin causing rashes, e.g. erythema marginatum.
5. Acute congestion and pulmonary oedema caused by the acute heart failure, secondary to the myocardial involvement.

87 1. Valvular heart disease, causing stenosis, incompetence or both.
2. Atrial fibrillation which predisposes to thrombus

formation in the atria (usually left) and their appendages. This may give rise to a 'ball-valve' thrombus or emboli.
3. Angina pectoris due to myocardial hypertrophy and decreased cardiac output, both caused by the valve disease.
4. Subacute bacterial endocarditis.

88 Chronic endocarditis is the term applied to the fibrosed, scarred and distorted valves which become stenosed, incompetent or both, following healing of acute rheumatic endocarditis. The condition is, therefore, not a chronic inflammatory disease, although occasional Aschoff bodies may be present in the myocardium.

89 An Aschoff body is a lesion, either of microscopic dimensions or just visible to the naked eye, which occurs in the myocardium in acute rheumatic fever. It is most commonly found in the interventricular septum, the left atrium and the left auricular appendage.

90 Aschoff bodies develop in the connective tissue septa adjacent to the small blood vessels within the myocardium. Each consists of a focus of 'fibrinoid necrosis' in the collagen associated with degeneration of a few myocardial fibres in the immediate vicinity. The cellular aggregation around each lesion chiefly consists of lymphocytes, plasmacytes and macrophages together with Aschoff cells. The last are large cells containing up to three pleomorphic nuclei. The lesion heals leaving a small scar.

91 Acute bacterial endocarditis is a fulminating condition associated with septicaemia caused by highly pathogenic organisms such as *Staphylococcus aureus*, occurring in an individual with a normal heart prior to the onset of the disease. It frequently occurs in addicts receiving their drugs by the intravenous route, in debilitated patients and in patients with a septic focus. Large friable vegetations develop on the heart valves which soon become ulcerated, fenestrated and distorted. The rapid destruction of the affected valve or valves, if unchecked, interferes with their function causing heart failure.

In contrast subacute bacterial endocarditis is caused by organisms of low pathogenicity including *Streptococcus viridans*, *Escherichia coli*, enterococci and occasionally fungi. The organism enters the bloodstream e.g. following tooth extraction or catheterisation, causing a bacteraemia rather than a septicaemia, and settles on valves already abnormal due to disease or suffering some congenital defect, e.g. a bicuspid aortic valve. Subacute bacterial endocarditis essentially presents as a low grade infection in which cure can nearly always be obtained by the administration of the correct antibiotic. If, however, vegetations have formed on the valves dysfunction nearly always results.

92 Infective endocarditis is divided for descriptive purposes into acute and subacute types although there is considerable overlap between them. The acute type is caused by virulent pathogenic organisms during the course of a septicaemia. Ulceration, fenestration and destruction of valves causes death. The subacute variety is most commonly caused by commensals or weak pathogens, classically *Streptococcus viridans* or by fungi in immunosuppressed patients. The endocardial infection is superimposed upon pre-existing disease, either a chronic endocarditis or some congenital malformation such as a bicuspid aortic valve, a septal defect or a patent ductus arteriosus.

93 1. Sudden death.
    2. Angina pectoris.
    3. Myocardial infarction.
    4. Cardiac failure due to myocardial fibrosis.
    5. Arrhythmias due to bundle branch block.

94 'Anguish in the chest'. A very severe pain in the chest usually on the left side frequently radiating into the left arm or into the neck or even the jaws and teeth. It is brought on by increase in cardiac output which, in turn, requires an increase in the myocardial blood flow to provide the necessary oxygen. It is relieved by rest or vasodilator drugs.

95 1. Immediate death due to heart failure due to cardiogenic shock.
    2. Early death due to rupture of the necrotic myocardium (myomalacia cordis), causing a haemopericardium.
    3. An arrhythmia.

4. A mural thrombus leading to embolic phenomena.
5. Chronic heart failure due to myocardial fibrosis.
6. Cardiac aneurysm.
7. Recovery followed by mild angina pectoris or no symptoms at all.

96 About 8 hours.

97 Arrhythmias such as atrial fibrillation, extrasystoles and paroxysmal tachycardia are not associated with specific pathological features. However, block of the AV bundle or its branches is frequently seen to be caused by:
1. myocardial infarction or ischaemic fibrosis
2. surgical trauma
3. a tumour
4. idiopathic fibrosis
Sometimes no morphologic changes are found in cases of heart block but since the structures affected are small and the changes may be slight, they are probably overlooked by the pathologist.

98 1. Rheumatic fever.
2. Suppurative myocarditis caused either by extension of a bacterial infection from the valves in an infective endocarditis or by haematogenous spread in the course of a septicaemia or pyaemia.
3. Viral myocarditis caused by the Coxsackie A or B viruses.
4. Sarcoidosis.
5. Syphilitic, the *Spirochaeta pallidum* may cause a variety of cardiac lesions:
   a. aortic incompetence
   b. myocardial ischaemia from narrowing of the coronary ostia
   c. gumma of the myocardium which may cause heart block if the conducting system is involved
   d. fibrosis of the myocardium due to miliary gummata in congenital syphilis
6. Toxic myocarditis resulting from an infective fever such as diphtheria, pneumococcal pneumonia or typhoid or any septicaemia
7. Isolated myocarditis for which there is no known cause, but it resembles viral myocarditis.

99 The term cardiomyopathy embraces many

unrelated chronic conditions of the myocardium whose causes are unknown. There are four types:
1. hypertrophic; in some patients this condition is inherited as an autosomal dominant gene. The myocardium is hypertrophied; microscopically the myocardial fibres are arranged in a typical whorled pattern. The thickening of the left ventricle interferes with systole and the thickened interventricular septum obstructs the outflow from the ventricles, affecting the left rather than the right. This type presents with angina or heart failure.
2. congestive; the myocardium is flabby and the various chambers of the heart dialated. Mural thrombi, together with endocardial and interstitial fibrosis may be present. Clinically the patient presents with congestive heart failure for which no cause can be found.
3. restrictive or endomyocardial fibro-elastosis; this is rare condition occurring in infancy in which a thick subendocardial layer of fibro-elastic tissue develops, chiefly in the left ventricle.
4. obliterative; this condition occurs chiefly in adults in tropical Africa. The endocardium is very fibrosed in the region of the papillary muscles and chordae tendinae.

100 An acutely failing heart may present as:
1. pulmonary oedema, due to left ventricular failure
2. cardiogenic shock due to a low output state
3. right heart failure in a right sided infarction or pulmonary embolism

Chronic heart failure. The presentation of chronic heart failure depends upon the side of the heart which is affected:
1. left sided; in most patients it is due to:
   a. ischaemic heart disease
   b. systemic hypertension
   c. aortic and mitral valve disease
   d. cardiomyopathies
   e. congenital heart disease

An early sign is dyspnoea on exertion progressing to dyspnoea at rest.
2. right sided; the common causes are:
   a. pulmonary hypertension from whatever cause, e.g. mitral stenosis, pulmonary fibrosis and thrombo-embolic disease
   b. tricuspid and pulmonary stenosis

These conditions produce hypertrophy followed by dilatation of the right side of the heart. The neck veins become dilated and there is evidence of venous congestion of the liver and spleen which may become palpable. Stasis predisposes to atrial thrombosis and pulmonary embolic phenomena.

101 1. Causes in the myocardium and pericardium:
   a. myocardial fibrosis caused by ischaemic heart disease
   b. myocarditis and the cardiomyopathies
   c. arrhythmias
   d. amyloidosis
   e. cardiac tamponade due to pericardial effusion or haemopericardium
   f. constrictive pericarditis
2. Increase in vascular resistance:
   a. systemic hypertension
   b. pulmonary hypertension
3. Increase in blood volume
   A regurgitant valve causes a volume overload which is followed by hypertrophy and later dilatation.
4. Pressure overload.
   A stenotic valve causes a proximal increase in pressure followed by gross hypertrophy and later failure.
5. Increase blood flow:
   a. a shunt between the left and right sides of the heart caused by atrio-ventricular septal defects or peripheral arteriovenous shunts as in Paget's disease of bone
   b. anaemia, thyrotoxicosis and beri-beri

102 In primary (essential or idiopathic hypertension), there is no known cause. In secondary, in the majority of patients the cause is chronic renal disease. Less common causes include primary aldosteronism, Cushing's syndrome or a phaeochromocytoma.

103 1. Left ventricular hypertrophy.
2. Vascular changes in:
   a. the large arteries. The earliest changes consists of hypertrophy of the smooth muscle and elastic fibres. Later fibrosis occurs so that the vessel wall is weakened although thickened.
   b. the small arteries. The changes in the smaller arteries of 1 mm or less in diameter

depend upon the type of hypertension i.e. whether it is benign or malignant. In the former, gross intimal thickening develops together with a lesser degree of medial thickening. In the latter, fibrinoid necrosis of the wall together with superadded thrombosis occurs.

104 1. Non-infective:
   a. acute rheumatic fever
   b. myocardial infarction
   c. metastatic tumours
   d. primary mesothelioma
   e. uraemia
2. Infective:
   a. pyogenic
   b. tuberculosis
   c. viral

105 Embarrassment of the heart's action by blood or other substance such as serous effusion or pus in the pericardial sac. This prevents diastolic filling. The condition is similar to constrictive pericarditis.

RESPIRATORY SYSTEM

106 1. Thrombi from the pelvic or iliac veins or deep veins of the leg.
2. Tumour, derived from primary tumours elsewhere in the body.
3. Fat, following fractures or merely trauma.
4. Marrow, following fractures.

107 No. Atelectasis means that the lung has never expanded from birth. Collapse occurs in a previously expanded lung and may be due to pressure (pressure collapse) or obstruction of a bronchus (absorption collapse).

108 Classically from the onset of the disease to healing, lobar pneumonia passes through four stages, each stage blending into the next.
1. Congestion. The alveolar capillaries are distended with blood.
2. Red hepatisation. Oedema fluid, erythrocytes and pus cells pass from the capillaries into the alveolar spaces in which fibrin is deposited. The lobe is consolidated.
3. Grey hepatisation. The congestion disappears partly due to capillary compression by the

intense cellular infiltration, which now includes macrophages, into the alveoli.
4. Resolution. The alveolar exudate is liquefied by enzymes liberated from the lysed inflammatory cells and is expectorated. Macrophages appear and engulf cellular debris and pneumococci.

109 1. Direct spread of the organism from the lung causing either a pleural effusion followed by an empyema or more rarely suppurative pericarditis.
2. Haematogenous spread leading to suppurative arthritis or meningitis.
3. Failure of resolution followed by organisation of the exudate. This process is known as carnification because of the solid, fleshy appearance of the fibrosed lung tissue.

110 Lobar pneumonia usually occurs in otherwise healthy young adults and in 90 per cent of cases is caused by *Streptococcus pneumoniae* whereas bronchopneumonia, due to the extension of a bronchitis or bronchiolitis, is most frequent in individuals whose resistance to infection has been reduced e.g. in infancy, by old age or by a debilitating condition such as malignancy or by malnutrition. In bronchopneumonia, a variety of organisms is responsible, usually commensals from the upper respiratory tract, such as the *Staphylococcus aureus*, *Streptococcus pyogenes* and *Haemophilus influenzae*. Lobar pneumonia may affect a part of a lobe, an entire lobe or several lobes, the affected areas passing through four distinct pathological changes whereas bronchopneumonia, otherwise known as lobular pneumonia, begins with mucosal damage in the small bronchioles and the acute inflammatory process affects the lobules they supply. Even before chemotherapy lobar pneumonia usually resolved spontaneously with no residual damage. Occasionally death due to respiratory failure, septicaemia or complications would occur. Untreated bronchopneumonia may result in varying degrees of fibrosis of the lung.

111 1. It is not caused by a pyogenic organism and the cellular response to the infection is therefore mononuclear i.e. lymphocytic, plasmacytic and histiocytic rather than polymorphonuclear.

2. The capsule of the organism contains mucoprotein and the sputum of the patient and the cut surface of the lung at autopsy are very mucoid.
3. There is usually much lung destruction, whereas resolution is the rule in other lobar pneumonias.

112
1. The inflammation is usually interstitial, the inflammatory response occurring in the walls of the alveoli rather than in the air spaces.
2. The cellular response is mononuclear.
3. In severe cases haemorrhage and necrosis occurs in the lung parenchyma.
4. Proliferation of the bronchiolar and alveolar epithelial cells occurs.
5. The disease is frequently fulminating.

113 Bronchiectasis, not chronic bronchitis.

114 Bronchiectasis means dilatation of the bronchi. It is seen following:
1. non-specific chronic inflammation of the bronchi
2. recurrent acute inflammation
3. obstruction of a bronchus

Why these conditions should cause bronchial dilatation is not known with certainty but the following factors are thought to be important:
1. inflammatory destruction of the bronchial walls causing loss of the smooth muscle and cartilage, thus weakening the walls
2. the pull of the elastic tissue in the alveolar walls on the external surface of the bronchi whose walls are weakened as above
3. interference with the nerve supply to the smooth muscle

115
1. Empyema and suppurative pericarditis
2. Pyaemia with the production of abscesses in other organs—notably brain
3. Amyloidosis
4. Cor pulmonale due to destruction of lung tissue

116 *Pneumocystis carinii* is a sporozoon. The reservoir is the rodent and infection in man is opportunistic. The affected lungs are uniformly consolidated and dry. The characteristic histological appearance is of foamy, fibrillary material in the

alveolar spaces. The organism forms cysts in the alveolar septal cells and the trophozoites, after proliferating in the cysts, are discharged into the alveoli. They can be demonstrated in the exudate by the use of PAS, Giemsa's or Gomori's (silver) stains.

117 Aspergillosis is manifest in three ways.
1. Non-invasive:
   a. allergic bronchopulmonary aspergillosis—an asthmatic condition
   b. mycetoma—a ball of the fungus growing in a preformed cavity in the lung, such as an old abscess, without invading the lung
2. Invasive, where the fungus infiltrates the lung parenchyma. This infection is usually opportunistic.

118 Empyema or pyothorax is pus in the pleural cavity and therefore implies infection by a pyogenic organism. Infection may occur from:
1. the lung as a complication of pneumonia
2. the chest wall following injury
3. the abdomen—extension of a subphrenic abscess
4. a perforated oesophagus and mediastinitis
5. blood spread (rarely)

119 1. Air
2. Serous effusion
3. Blood-stained effusion
4. Pus
5. Chyle
6. Blood

120 1. Haemodynamic and osmotic; due to heart failure or hypoproteinaemia as in liver failure or malnutrition
2. Inflammatory; serous, sero-purulent and haemorrhagic effusions and empyema
3. Neoplasms; serous or haemorrhagic effusions
4. Obstruction to or tearing of the thoracic duct; chylothorax

121 1. Fibrogenic, usually caused by inorganic dusts, e.g. anthraco-silicosis or silicosis, asbestosis, berylliosis and various other metallic dusts whose fumes may also cause an acute chemical pneumonia
2. Allergic, usually due to organic dusts, e.g.

bagassosis (sugar cane waste), byssinosis (cotton), farmer's lung (thermophilic actinomycetes), bird fancier's lung (protein in birds' droppings)

122 Interstitial fibrosis of the lungs associated with the development of fibrous pleural plaques. Less common is the induction of pleural and sometimes peritoneal mesotheliomata by blue asbestos (crocidolite). Asbestos also potentiates the carcinogenic effect on the lung of cigarette smoking, but alone it is only a mild lung carcinogen.

123 Emphysema is an enlargement of the air spaces of the lung accompanied by destruction of alveolar walls. In overinflation there is no destruction and this condition is therefore reversible although it will progress to emphysema if it becomes chronic.

124 1. Generalised:
   a. centriacinar (also called centrilobular or bronchiolar, the respiratory bronchiole being involved)
   b. panacinar
   c. paraseptal
2. Bullous emphysema is applied to advanced cases of 1. but an occasional single bulla may be present in young people. If it ruptures, spontaneous pneumothorax or interstitial (surgical) emphysema may occur.
3. Paratractional, when the emphysema occurs round shrunken scars or silicotic nodes
4. Compensatory, in a lobe or lobes when another lobe or a lung has collapsed or has been excised
5. Senile

125 Chronic bronchitis has a clinical definition (chronic cough with sputum production on most days during a 3 month period of the year for at least two years in succession). It does not mean chronic inflammation of bronchi. There are therefore no pathognomonic features but the following are likely to be seen in the bronchi histologically:
1. an increase in the bronchial goblet cells at the expense of the ciliated epithelium (mucous metaplasia)
2. hypertrophy of the submucosal mucous glands
3. the changes of non-specific acute bronchitis if there is superadded inflammation

4. emphysema, which is frequently associated with chronic bronchitis

126 Grossly, the lungs are overinflated and do not collapse when the chest is opened. Section reveals tough mucus plugs filling the bronchi. Microscopically the following are seen:
1. mucus plugs in bronchi containing many eosinophils together with Curschmann's spirals (characteristic coils of mucin) and Charcot-Leyden crystals, derived from the granules of eosinophils
2. an excess of goblet cells in the bronchial epithelium
3. hypertrophy of the submucosal mucus glands in bronchi
4. non-specific acute bronchitis if superadded infection had occurred

127 A condition leading to respiratory distress in premature infants due to lack of surfactant, a lipoprotein produced by type 2 pneumocytes. The hyaline membrane which lines the alveolar walls is composed of fibrin and degenerating cells. Exposure to high oxygen concentrations may be a contributory factor. Surfactant is a detergent-like substance which, decreasing surface tension, normally prevents alveolar collapse.

128 There are two main varieties, the childhood and the adult respiratory distress syndromes. Both are clinical conditions having various causes. The former is usually due to hyaline membrane disease but can be caused by overzealous treatment with oxygen. The latter is an end-stage, or fibrosed lung, resulting from numerous diverse agents among which are the inhalation of a high concentration of oxygen during resuscitation, paraquat poisoning, shock, x-irradiation or unresolved pneumonia. The basic pathology in all of the above appears to be oedema into the alveolar walls and air spaces with fibrin deposition in both. The fibrin finally organises into scar tissue which thickens the walls and fills the alveoli.

129 1. Cigarette smoking is the most significant factor. Cigar and pipe smoking have been incriminated but to a lesser extent.
2. Exposure to crocidolite, one of the three types of asbestos. Alone the inhalation of crocidolite

causes only a modest increase in the incidence of lung cancer but it potentiates the carcinogenic effect of cigarette smoking considerably.

3. In the past the inhalation of radioactive dusts and gases by the miners of various metal ores in Czechoslovakia and Saxony was an important occupational hazard.

130 Lung cancers may be primary bronchogenic carcinomata or secondary (metastatic) growths from elsewhere. Lymphomata and leukaemias are included in the latter although primary lymphomata of lung do occur. Bronchogenic carcinomata may possess a heterogeneous structure; they are classified histologically.

Histological classifications vary slightly but most growths can be placed in one of the following categories:
1. squamous (epidermoid) carcinomata
2. oat cell (small cell or anaplastic) carcinomata
3. adenocarcinomata
4. anaplastic (large cell anaplastic) carcinomata
5. broncho-alveolar carcinomata

The last may be a variety of adenocarcinoma or, as some consider, they may be derived from the alveolar epithelium, in which case they are lung, rather than bronchogenic, carcinomata.

131 The cells of an oat-cell carcinoma usually contain neurosecretory granules as shown by the electron microscope and the tumour sometimes produces the carcinoid syndrome which suggests that the origin of the growth is from APUD (Feyrter) cells. Although this accounts for 5-HT secretion by some of these tumours, others appear to secrete different hormones, e.g. ADH and ACTH.

HAEMATOLOGY

132 A measure of the maturity or age of neutrophil polymorphs assessed by counting the numbers of lobes in their nuclei. The number with a non-lobulated (one lobed) nucleus is placed on the left of a table and those with increasing numbers of lobes up to 5 are progressively inserted to the right. A 'shift to the right' means there are more multilobulated nuclei, i.e. older cells whilst the converse means the polymorphs are newly shed from the marrow.

133
1. Hypersensitivity states such as hay fever and urticaria
2. Infections by animal parasites, notably helminths such as trichinella and schistosoma
3. Certain chronic skin diseases; pemphigus and pemphigoid
4. Some patients with polyarteritis nodosa
5. Some cases of Hodgkin's lymphoma

134
1. Haematology:
   a. Moderate reduction in RBC count
   b. Relatively greater reduction in haemoglobin; the MCHC is most significant, about 25–30 g/dl
   c. White cell and platelet counts are normal
   d. Slight or moderate normoblastic hyperplasia of marrow
   e. Iron stores depleted in the reticuloendothelial system
2. Biochemistry:
   a. Low plasma iron
   b. Normal or low plasma bilirubin
3. General pathology:
   The changes occur essentially in epithelia and appendages in chronic cases
   a. Mouth—angular stomatitis
   b. Tongue—atrophy of filiform papillae
   c. Hypopharynx—Plummer-Vinson (Paterson-Kelly) syndrome
   d. Stomach mucosa may atrophy as in megaloblastic anaemia
   e. Koilonychia
   f. Alopecia

135 This was first described by Paterson and Kelly who noted an association between iron-deficiency anaemia, glossitis and dysphagia with atrophy of the pharyngeal muscles and a pharyngeal web with stricture formation, in middle-aged women. A post-cricoid squamous carcinoma frequently developed later. The reason for this association is obscure.

136
1. Haemolytic anaemias are due to defects in the erythrocytes:
   a. hereditary spherocytosis
   b. hereditary elliptocytosis
   c. enzyme deficiencies such as pyruvate kinase deficiency
2. The haemoglobinopathies:

a. sickle cell disease
   b. the thalassaemias
   c. paroxysmal nocturnal haemoglobinuria
3. Changes outside the cell:
   a. the presence of autoantibodies. Most are idiopathic but some develop in response to infection or the presence of malignancy
   b. the presence of alloantibodies, the commonest of which is the rhesus factor
   c. drugs
   d. toxins, e.g. the haemolysin produced by *Streptococcus haemolyticus*
4. Infection of the red cell, e.g. by the malaria parasite
5. Mechanical trauma:
   a. the presence of a heart valve prosthesis
   b. cardiopulmonary bypass
   c. disseminated intravascular coagulation causing the deposition of small strands of fibrin in the small blood vessels

137 Pigment gall stones are caused by supersaturation and precipitation in the bile of excess bile pigment derived from lysed erythrocytes.

138 There is a tendency for haemolysis, which occurs in almost all anaemias whether haemolytic or not.

139 Deficiency of Vitamin B_{12} or folic acid or both. Rarely defective DNA synthesis. These occur in:
1. famine
2. chronic atrophic gastritis which is possibly an autoimmune condition, causing deficiency of intrinsic factor
3. malabsorption by the intestine (e.g. ileal by-pass, Crohn's disease)
4. pregnancy (increased requirements with inadequate diet)
5. cirrhosis of liver (disordered folate metabolism or inadequate intake)
6. fish tapeworm (*Diphyllobothrium latum*) infestation
7. increased erythropoiesis as in haemolytic anaemias
8. DNA synthesis disturbance; inherited disorders or due to treatment with cytotoxic drugs

140 1. Haematology:
       a. Low RBC count

b. Low Hb. concentration
   c. Increased MCV and MCH
   d. MCHC normal
   e. The erythrocytes show macrocytosis, anisocytosis, poikilocytosis and polychromasia
   f. Neutropaenia and thrombocytopaenia
   g. Megaloblastic and myeloid hyperplasia
2. Biochemistry:
   a. Slight raised plasma bilirubin, 17–51 mmol/l (1–3 mg/dl)
   b. Urobilinuria
   c. Increased urobilinogen in faeces
   d. Raised plasma iron
   e. Achlorhydria in pernicious anaemia and occasionally in other megaloblastic anaemias
3. General pathology:
   a. Fatty degeneration of heart, liver and kidneys
   b. Haemosiderosis of kidneys and liver parenchymal cells and spleen and marrow reticuloendothelial cells.
   c. Subacute combined degeneration of the spinal cord is seen as demyelination of the lateral and posterior columns. There is no gliosis
   d. Atrophy of tongue (the filiform papillae) and gastric mucosa in pernicious anaemia
   e. Extension of the red marrow (hyperplasia) along shafts of long bones

141 Failure of haemopoiesis. Malignant infiltration of the marrow is excluded. Usually all elements of the marrow are involved. The common variety is idiopathic aplastic anaemia for which no cause can be found. Known causes of the condition are:
1. infection, e.g. miliary TB
2. drugs, especially cytotoxic agents
3. irradiation
4. hypopituitarism

142 1. Lymphatic:
      a. acute lymphatic (acute lymphoblastic)
      b. chronic lymphatic
   2. Myeloid:
      a. acute myeloid (acute myeloblastic)
      b. chronic myeloid
      The affected cell is nearly always the neutrophil but chronic eosinophilic and basophilic leukaemias have been described rarely.
   3. Monocytic (uncommon):

     a. acute monocytic (acute monoblastic)
     b. chronic monocytic
Since the monocyte and granulocyte have a common stem cell, the acute monocytic may have features of acute myeloid when the variety, acute monomyeloblastic is recognised.

143 Polycythaemia is a state in which there is an increase in the number of red cells in the blood together with an increase in the blood volume.

    Primary polycythaemia, also known as polycythaemia vera, is a neoplastic condition of the erythroid series.

    Secondary polycythaemia is a physiological response, usually to hypoxia. It therefore occurs in:
a. individuals living at high altitudes
b. patients suffering from chronic pulmonary disease
c. congenital cyanotic cardiac conditions

It may, however, also occur in Cushing's disease and in malignancy if the primary tumour secretes an erythropoietin-like factor.

144 1. The red cells are normocytic and normochromic
    2. The patient is plethoric
    3. Splenomegaly and hepatomegaly occur due to extramedullary haemopoiesis
    4. Tendency to thrombosis is due to increased blood viscosity and thrombocythaemia
    5. Inexplicable haemorrhages may occur
    6. Occasional conversion to myeloid leukaemia or myelofibrosis with anaemia

145 An unusual condition in which the haemopoietic marrow is replaced by fibrous tissue or, occasionally an overgrowth of the adjacent bone. The last is described as osteosclerosis when seen on x-ray. Extra-medullary haemopoiesis occurs in liver, spleen and other organs and since it may predate the marrow destruction, the disease is considered to be a myeloproliferative disorder, especially since it has much in common with polycythaemia vera. It tends to be more chronic than myeloid leukaemia and may be related to it.

146 Purpura is a condition in which there is bleeding into the skin and/or mucous membranes. Haemorrhages less than 2 mm in diameter are called petechiae and when larger, ecchymoses. In neither

is the skin raised, if it is, the lesion is a haematoma.

147 Factor III (thromboplastin) which is part of the extrinsic pathway of the clotting mechanism. When absent, thrombin formation occurs very slowly. Injury to the vascular endothelium or endocardium by allowing the entry of Factor III into the blood causes intravascular thrombosis.

Within the blood itself there are also a variety of inhibitors including:
1. several antithrombins, the most important of which are:
   a. fibrin, which when deposited in the blood in small amounts, filters thrombin out of the blood stream
   b. antithrombin III, a heparin co-factor
2. heparin which acts through co-factors such as 1.b. above

148 1. Platelet abnormalities:
   Thrombocytopaenia due to:
   a. destruction as in idiopathic thrombocytopaenic purpura
   b. increased consumption, as in disseminated intravascular coagulation or thrombotic thrombocytopaenic purpura
   c. failure of production as in aplastic anaemia and marrow replacement by cancer
   d. miscellaneous causes including infections, drugs, massive transfusions of blood whose platelets are effete
2. Damage to capillaries:
   a. Henoch-Schönlein purpura
   b. Scurvy
   c. Infections, e.g. meningococcal septicaemia
   d. Drugs
3. Defects in clotting mechanisms—usually hereditary:
   a. Haemophilia
   b. Haemophilia B (Christmas disease)
   c. Von Willebrand's disease
   d. Other rare conditions where various specific clotting factors are deficient

149 1. Fibrinogen synthesis is reduced in severe liver failure.
2. The defibrination syndrome. This occurs in two ways:
   a. the fibrinolytic syndrome due to activation

of the plasmin system. This can occur during major operations and also in patients with severe liver or congenital heart disease. Plasmin can be detected in the blood and it degrades fibrin and other clotting factors. Bleeding, with a normal platelet count, are the main features. Fibrin degradation products (FDP) are found in the blood.
b. Disseminated intravascular coagulation (DIC) is due to clotting factors released into the blood and/or severe damage to endothelium. Fibrinogen is converted to fibrin intravascularly. Platelets are involved so thrombocytopaenia occurs. Both haemorrhage and infarction due to small thrombi occur in this condition. There are numerous causes such as incomplete blood transfusion, abruptio placentae, severe trauma, major operations, fat embolism and severe infections.

150 A fragmented red cell which takes the form of a triangle, crescent or microspherocyte. It is the result of physical trauma to the red cell and occurs when a cardiac prosthesis such as a Borg valve has been inserted. The fragmentation is a form of haemolysis and results in anaemia. Schistocytes are also found in disseminated intravascular coagulation when the strands of fibrin which are deposited in the vessels are believed to cause the fragmentation.

LYMPHATIC SYSTEM

151 Enlargement due to stimulation as a result of lymph draining into it, usually from a chronically infected part. The sinuses may be distended by lymph containing numerous macrophages as well as lymphocytes and possibly polymorphs. These appearances are described as 'sinus catarrh'. In addition, there may be hyperplasia and hypertrophy of lymphoid follicles with their germinal centres. Chronic irritation as a result of an itchy skin lesion or even drainage from a cancer, without metastasis being present in the node, may cause reactive hyperplasia.

152 1. Congenital absence or aplasia of the lymphatics, Milroy's disease

2. Neoplastic permeation
3. Chronic lymphangitis
4. Invasion of the lymphatics by *Wuchereria bancrofti*, the adult worm blocking the lymphatics, particularly those draining lower limbs and genitalia

153 Multinucleate giant cells seen in lymphoid tissue in cases of measles.

154 Glandular fever or infectious mononucleosis is caused by infection with a virus, almost certainly the Epstein-Barr virus. Although it is an infectious condition it is not highly contagious; kissing is considered to be a common mode of transmission. The virus probably enters the epithelial cells of the pharynx and infects B lymphocytes which are transformed, permitting their indefinite culture *in vitro*. They thus resemble Burkitt lymphoma cells but infectious mononucleosis does not predispose to lymphomas. *In vivo*, the virus replicates in B lymphocytes and infects others. T cell response also occurs and these T immunoblasts, being cytotoxic, limit the infection and proliferation of B cells, which, it is considered, would otherwise constitute a neoplasm. The T cell cytotoxicity is responsible for the necrosis of the infected pharyngeal epithelial cells and secondary infection causes a severe suppurative pharyngitis and tonsillitis with pyrexia. Lymph node architecture is not destroyed but the nodes enlarge due to reactive hyperplasia and contain large atypical blast cells which may suggest lymphoma. These are the T cells which are almost diagnostic when seen in a blood film. Being larger than normal lymphocytes, they were originally considered to be monocytes when seen in the blood, hence the name of the disease. A leucocytosis of 10 to 20 $\times 10^9$/l occurs due to the presence of these cells. The disease is self-limiting after some weeks. Hepatitis, with jaundice occurs occasionally. A reliable diagnostic test for this disease is the Paul-Bunnell which detects the heterophil agglutinins that develop in most patients to sheep red cells. Syphilis is occasionally responsible for a false positive Paul-Bunnell test.

155 Three uncommon conditions fall into this category. They are of unknown aetiology and are typified by neoplastic-like proliferations of macro-

phages but are not considered neoplasms. The conditions are:
1. Letterer-Siwe disease, which is rapidly fatal and affects children. It is essentially due to marrow replacement by macrophages which do not contain lipid.
2. Hand-Schuller-Christian disease sometimes affects adults but mostly occurs in children and the macrophages contain lipids, mainly cholesterol. The patient may survive up to ten years. Lipid accumulation is not the cause of this disease and it is therefore not a lipid-storage disease.
3. Eosinophil granuloma of bone. This is a solitary lesion and possibly represents an indolent variety of Letterer-Siwe in which eosinophils accompany the collections of macrophages. It occurs in adolescents and young adults.

156 A malignant condition of lymphatic tissue excluding thymoma and leukaemia. It may present primarily in a lymph node or group of nodes or in the spleen, thymus, or indeed, any site where lymphoid tissue is present e.g. marrow or the wall of the stomach or intestine. Lymphoma may also arise primarily in the skin—mycosis fungoides. The disease eventually becomes multifocal or at least the malignant lymphocytes invade the body widely and, in the case of non-Hodgkin's lymphoma, may spill into the blood stream to cause lymphatic leukaemia.

157 The Kiel classification in current international use is as follows:
1. those of low malignancy:
   a. lymphocytic
   b. centrocytic
   c. centroblastic-centrocytic, which can be follicular, diffuse or mixed
2. those of high malignancy:
   a. lymphoblastic which includes Burkitt's lymphoma
   b. centroblastic
   c. immunoblastic

There is also an Unclassified Group in each of 1 and 2.

158 The Reed-Sternberg cell is an essential feature of Hodgkin's disease. It is large, 40 μm or more in diameter, and characteristically has a bilobed

nucleus and abundant eosinophilic cytoplasm which is sometimes vacuolated.

159 The Ann Arbor system of staging.
Stage I: one node or a group of nodes is affected
Stage II: the affected nodes are either all above or all below the diaphragm
Stage III: nodes both above and below the diaphragm are affected with or without lesions in other tissues
Stage IV: there is widespread involvement of one or more non-lymphoid tissues with or without nodal involvement.

The importance is for treatment and prognosis. A single node or group (Stages I and II) is treated by local radiotherapy. Otherwise chemotherapy is given. As well as the histological type the stage affects the prognosis; the higher the stage, the poorer the outlook.

160 By histological appearances and, at present, the Rye classification is internationally agreed. The following four groups are recognised:
1. lymphocyte-predominant, where most cells are lymphocytes, Reed-Sternberg cells are frequent and eosinophils are very scanty.
2. lymphocyte-depleted. Many Reed-Sternberg cells with variable eosinophils are present. Fibrosis may be prominent but is diffuse. Lymphocytes are sparse.
3. nodular sclerosing where the capsule is thickened by collagen which sends trabeculae through the node
4. mixed cellularity. Reed-Sternberg cells, macrophages, neutrophils, eosinophils, lymphocytes and plasmacytes are all present. There may be diffuse (unlike 3.) collagen.

Fifteen per cent of cases of Hodgkin's disease fall into each of groups 1. and 2. and 30 to 40 per cent into each of 3. and 4. Nodular sclerosis in Stage I of the disease has the best prognosis. Otherwise lymphocyte-predominant has the best prognosis, mixed cellularity is worse and lymphocyte-depleted the worst. The disease tends to progress in the order of the last three.

Although prognosis is related to the above types, treatment is determined by the stage only.

161 This is a malignant lymphoma which occurs in the

skin. The upper dermis is infiltrated by macrophages, lymphocytes, reticulum cells, plasma cells and eosinophil leucocytes. Collections of lymphocytes, the Pautrier's abscesses, are found in the epidermis.

162 Splenomegaly is enlargement of the spleen from any cause. The commonest cause globally is probably malaria. In Britain, portal hypertension is responsible for most cases. An enlarged spleen predisposes to an increase of normal splenic activity regarding sequestration and destruction of elements of the blood and this is described as hypersplenism. Thus normocytic anaemia, leucopaenia and thrombocytopaenia develop. In some cases, hypersplenism occurs due to primary splenomegaly, i.e. there is no known reason for the enlarged spleen. Congestive splenomegaly usually due to portal hypertension with the above features of hypersplenism (mainly anaemia) is described as Banti's syndrome.

163 1. Infections:
   a. pyogenic
   b. non-pyogenic:
      (i) typhoid
      (ii) brucellosis
      (iii) tuberculosis
      (iv) protozoal—malaria or kala-azar
2. Neoplasms:
   a. leukaemias of any type. Massive enlargement occurs in chronic myeloid leukaemia and chronic lymphocytic leukaemia
   b. lymphomata:
      (i) Hodgkin's
      (ii) non-Hodgkin's
3. Haematological disorders:
   a. haemolytic anaemia
   b. macrocytic anaemia
   c. extra-medullary haemopoiesis
4. Portal hypertension from any cause
5. Amyloidosis
6. Lipid storage disorders:
   a. Gaucher's disease
   b. Niemann-Pick disease
7. Histiocytosis X
8. Cysts:
   a. following trauma
   b. echinococcal

164   1. Hyperlipidaemias
     2. Hereditary diseases
       a. In Gaucher's disease, which is uncommon, glucocerebrosides accumulate in macrophages (Gaucher cells) in various organs. The disease is due to an autosomal recessive gene and the heterozygous carrier can be identified by demonstrating beta-glucuronidase deficiency in macrophages. The lack of this enzyme results in the accumulation of the lipid.
       b. Niemann-Pick disease is rare. The phospholipid, sphingomyelin, together with other lipids such as cholesterol are found in macrophages which infiltrate spleen, liver, marrow, nodes, brain, endocrine glands etc. An autosomal recessive gene is probably responsible. The disease is manifest in early childhood as mental deficiency and is rapidly fatal.

166 They are organised infarcts of varying size in the spleen found most commonly in patients suffering from portal hypertension. They are composed of siderotic nodules consisting of collagenous fibrous tissue, fibroblasts and histiocytes. There is also considerable extracellular and intracellular haemosiderin and dystrophic calcification.

166 Rarely. The thymomata are the commonest. These tumours may be encapsulated and benign or locally infiltrative. They have a variable microscopic appearance containing both epithelial and lymphocytic elements. Thymomata are sometimes associated with myasthenia gravis. The other primary tumours of this gland are teratomata and lymphomata. Secondary growths from other sites are rare.

MOUTH AND SALIVARY GLANDS

167 Painful fissuring at the angles of the mouth. Loss of teeth and fold formation with age, causing irritation by saliva, may predispose but nutritional deficiencies (B vitamins and iron) play a part. Candida and staphylococcal infections may occur.

168 Recurrent oral ulcers which may be due to dietary

deficiencies (B vitamins or iron) or food allergies. In many cases no cause can be found.

169 1. Painful infection of the mouth, mainly gums, with ulceration and necrosis. Two commensal symbiotic organisms are present in large numbers but whether they cause the condition or form an overgrowth as a result of it is not known. They are *Fusobacterium fusiforme* and *Borrelia vincenti*.
2. Cellulitis of the floor of the mouth and neck causing severe oedema due to a spreading haemolytic streptococcal infection. It usually arises from a tonsillitis. As the names suggest, both conditions cause anxiety.

170 Salivary calculi are composed of calcium carbonate and calcium phosphate. They are commonest in the submandibular gland and its duct and rarely occur in the parotid. Obstruction of the duct predisposes to infection and possibly abscess formation. Repeated attacks of subacute inflammation and obstruction lead to atrophy and fibrosis of the affected salivary gland.

171 The fundamental pathological feature of Sjögren's syndrome, which is commoner in women than in men, is destruction of the salivary and lacrimal glands, with enlargement due to lymphocytic infiltration. Clinically the destruction of these glands results in dryness of the mouth causing difficulty in eating, and kerato-conjunctivitis sicca. Associated with these changes may be lymphadenoid goitre. Auto-antibodies to the microsomal fraction of all these glands may be present.

172 Sarcoidosis causing iridocyclitis and parotitis.

173 1. Normal melanin in a coloured person
2. Excessive melanin in Addison's disease
3. Patchy pigmentation in the mouth and circumoral skin in the Peutz-Jeghers syndrome
4. Metallic poisons. Typically lead poisoning produces the 'lead line' on the gums at the neck of the teeth. This is caused by the formation of lead sulphide by bacterial action.

174 Leukoplakia is a clinical term indicating the presence of white patches in the mucosa of the mouth,

larynx, vulva or penis. There is a variety of causes, irritation due to smoking, carcinoma-in-situ, fungal infection or lichen planus. The whiteness of the mucosa is due to hyperkeratosis.

175 The pleomorphic salivary adenomata which constitute about 70% of salivary gland tumours occur mostly in the parotid gland where they are known as mixed parotid tumours. They can, however, arise in any gland, even in the minor glands of the mouth including gums and palate. They are essentially slow-growing, benign tumours but due to difficulty in complete excision, remaining islets of the growth are responsible for recurrences. Histologically, the tumour is composed of two elements in varying proportions, well-differentiated glandular structures and a stroma of spindle cells with much mucoid ground substance. Cartilage may occur in the latter. Complete excision is difficult due to the vulnerability of the facial nerve which ramifies through the gland. Malignant change is rare.

ALIMENTARY SYSTEM

176 Fungi seldom cause gastrointestinal disease in normal individuals. In debilitated or immunosuppressed people the following fungi may affect the gastrointestinal tract:
  1. the mucorales; *Mucor* and *Rhizopus*, which particularly affect the oesophagus and stomach
  2. *Candida albicans*, affecting particularly the oesophagus and stomach
  3. *Histoplasma*, usually affect the small gut

177 Dilatations of submucosal and subserosal veins which develop in patients suffering from portal obstruction. Although these venous plexuses normally drain into the systemic venous system, there are small anastomotic veins connecting them with the portal drainage of the stomach. High pressure in the portal system forces blood through the anastomoses into the systemic oesophageal veins which become dilated and varicose.

178 Reflux oesophagitis is usually associated with the sliding type of hiatus hernia. The reflux of the acidic gastric contents causes the development of oesophagitis and the symptom of severe heart-

burn. However, the severity of the heartburn is not reflected by the pathological changes in the oesophagus which may be mild.

179 1. Infiltration of the mucosa with lymphocytes, plasma cells and histiocytes
2. Hyperplasia of the basal cell layer of the squamous epithelium lining the oesophagus.
3. Loss of the more superficial cells bringing the connective tissue papillae of the lamina propria closer than normal to the surface
4. Ulceration followed by submucosal fibrosis which eventually may lead to stenosis and dysphagia

180 A Barrett's ulcer is a penetrating ulcer of the lower oesophagus, the oesophagus being lined by mucus-secreting instead of squamous epithelium. Such ulcers resemble peptic ulcers and may eventually lead to a severe bleeding or perforation.

181 The Mallory-Weiss syndrome consists of severe haemorrhage from a superficial tear of the wall of the lower end of the oesophagus or the cardia; the tear usually being caused by severe retching or a suppressed vomit.

182 1. Carcinoma
2. Peptic stricture
3. Achalasia
4. Rarer causes include:
   a. progressive 'systemic' sclerosis
   b. strictures caused by swallowing corrosives
   c. external compression due most commonly to malignant lymphadenopathy within the posterior mediastinum or an aneurysm of the aortic arch
   d. Chagas' disease caused by a protozoon, *Trypanosoma cruzi*, common in South America. This parasite exerts a toxic effect on the autonomic ganglia in various sites including the oesophagus

183 1. Squamous carcinoma which arises from the stratified squamous epithelium lining the oesophagus. Lesions of this type in the post cricoid region are some twenty times more common in women than in men.
2. Adenocarcinoma occurring at the lower end of

the oesophagus due to direct extension of tumours originating in the cardiac end of the stomach.

184 The commonest macroscopic appearance is of a raised nodule on the mucosa in the centre of which a variable degree of ulceration has occurred. Occasionally an annular growth occurs and even more rarely diffuse infiltration produces a long stricture. Microscopically the same tumour may have all grades of differentiation from a keratinsing squamous carcinoma exhibiting cell nests to an undifferentiated tumour in which neither keratin nor prickle cells are present.

185 1. Three-quarters of all squamous carcinomata of the oesophagus arise in the middle third.
2. In women, a squamous carcinoma may arise in the post-cricoid region as part of the Plummer-Vinson (Patterson-Kelly) syndrome

186 Carcinoma of the oesophagus spreads:
1. within the submucosal lymphatics to other parts of the oesophagus. This is particularly important to the surgeon because it may be unrecognised at operation only to be identified later at microscopy by the pathologist
2. via the lymphatics externally to the regional lymph nodes;
3. direct spread, after the muscular coats are breached, to involve the trachea, bronchi, lungs or posterior mediastinum
4. by the bloodstream to produce metastatic disease in the liver, lungs or adrenal glands

187 There are two types, the sliding type in which the gastro-oesophageal junction passes upwards into the thorax, and the para-oesophageal in which the gastro-oesophageal junction remains in its normal position and the fundus of the stomach passes upwards into the thorax. The chief fundamental difference between the two types is that, in the former, severe heartburn develops because incompetence of the gastro-oesophageal junction allows acid to enter the oesophagus, whereas the latter may be symptomless.

188 Erosions:
1. are frequently multiple
2. result from a loss of less than the full thickness

of the mucosa leaving some basal gland elements
3. usually heal without scarring

whereas an ulcer:
1. is a circumscribed lesion in which the full thickness of the mucosa is lost
2. has variable degrees of penetration of the underlying submucosa, muscularis mucosa and muscular layers
3. heals with scarring

189 By definition there is absence of the mucosa at the ulcer and the surrounding mucosa shows chronic inflammatory changes. The floor of the ulcer contains indeterminate necrotic material among which polymorphs may be recognised. Deep to this, the base of the ulcer, there is either active granulation tissue or mature collagen with fibroblasts, depending on the stage of activity or healing. The granulation tissue consists of newly developed capillaries lined by plump endothelial cells and contains inflammatory cells, scattered and in foci. These are mainly lymphocytes and plasma cells with some polymorphs. This granulation or fibrous tissue replaces all the normal coats of the stomach wall beneath the ulcer down to and including the muscularis propria, partly or entirely.

190 1. Perforation; either into the lesser sac, the general peritoneal cavity or perigastric tissues, notably the pancreas
2. Haemorrhage; into the stomach
3. Extensive fibrosis; leading to an 'hour-glass' stomach or pyloric stenosis
4. Cancer; this is controversial. It is never associated with duodenal ulcers but may account for approximately 1 per cent of gastric carcinomata.

191 1. Diet.
   a. Possibly pickled vegetables and dried salted fish. The latter is particularly important in Japan.
   b. Polycyclic hydrocarbons, significant in Iceland where much smoked mutton and trout are eaten.
2. Sex. The male/female ratio is unity in young adults, approaches 2:1 in the sixties and thereafter declines to unity in old age.
3. N-nitrosamines. These potent carcinogens are

produced by bacterial action on secondary amines, nitrates and nitrites. This factor may account for the increased incidence of cancer in the gastric remnant following gastrectomy.
4. Genetic factors. In the Caucasian there is a higher incidence of gastric cancer in people whose blood group is A.
5. Pernicious anaemia, possibly related to the associated mucosal atrophy.
6. Although 1 per cent of all gastric cancers arise in peptic ulcers it is not definitely known that the latter predisposes to the cancer.

192 This syndrome is caused by either a gastrin-secreting tumour of the islet cells of the pancreas or by hyperplasia of the antral gastrin-secreting cells.

The hypersecretion of gastrin causes:
1. hypersecretion of the gastric mucosa accompanied by the excessive secretion of hydrochloric acid
2. the rapid development of multiple peptic ulcers in the duodenum and upper jejunum

Secondary to the excessive secretion of acid, steatorrhoea or a watery diarrhoea may occur.

193 The term 'early gastric cancer' defines a gastric neoplasm which is confined to the mucosa or mucosa and submucosa. Lymphatic drainage from these may result in invasion of regional nodes even though the primary carcinoma seems small and localised.

194 Fifty per cent of all carcinomata of the stomach arise in the antrum and pyloric region. The second commonest site is in the cardia.

195 1. *Vibrio cholerae* causes cholera. Profuse fluid ('rice water') stools are passed containing small flakes of desquamated epithelium. Microscopy reveals desquamation and necrosis of the enterocytes particularly over the tips of the villi. Death occurs due to dehydration and hypokalaemia.
2. *Campylobacter* genus causes a profuse watery diarrhoea as with cholera but the infection is much less severe and is rarely fatal except in infants if hydration is not maintained.
3. *Escherichia coli*, strains A and B. Both cause severe diarrhoea in infancy and childhood with

gross dilatation of the gut. Microscopy reveals loss of the jejunal and ileal villi and oedema of the lamina propria. The mucosa is infiltrated by polymorphonuclear leucocytes among which the bacilli are seen.

4. *Staphylococcus aureus* causes severe diarrhoea in both infants and children. Gross mucosal ulceration occurs, deep to which is an acute inflammatory reaction.
5. *Salmonella typhi* causes typhoid fever with typical ulceration.
6. *Yersinia pseudotuberculosis* and *enterocolitica* chiefly affect children and young adults. They cause both mesenteric adenitis and lesions in the small bowel which, when exposed at laparotomy, resemble Crohn's disease macroscopically. Microscopically granulomata similar to caseating tubercles are seen in the gut wall and associated lymph nodes.

196 1. By direct spread, within the submucosa and muscle coats, occasionally accompanied by extensive fibrosis producing the condition known as 'linitis plastica' or 'leather bottle' stomach. Penetration of the serosa leads to the direct involvement of other parts of the gastrointestinal tract, notably the transverse colon.
2. By the lymphatics
3. By the bloodstream
4. Via the peritoneal cavity to produce peritoneal seedlings and ascites and occasionally tumours of the ovaries known as Krukenberg tumours

197 Giardiasis causes acute focal inflammation of the crypts of Lieberkuhn, principally in the duodenum and jejunum. Giardia are seldom found at the sites of inflammation although they are frequently present in the mucus between the villi and in the lamina propria and submucosa. The distortion caused by histological processing causes them to appear as sickle-shaped bodies which possess a basophilic cytoplasm and two nuclei. Giardiasis causes abdominal discomfort, distension, diarrhoea and lassitude. Fat absorption is disturbed and in children a sprue-like syndrome develops.

198 When a length of small bowel is resected the physiological effect is determined largely by the site of resection. An ileal resection always produces more severe malabsorption than a jejunal

because the terminal ileum can adapt to the loss of the jejunum, but not conversely. Following massive small gut resection the number of enterocytes per unit length of each villus increases.

199 A state of malabsorption caused by damage to the mucosa of the small bowel by a breakdown product of gluten to which the patient is sensitive. The chief histological feature is in the small bowel and removal of the gluten from the diet causes clinical improvement and some or total return to anatomical normality.

200 1. Shortening in height and an increase in the width of small bowel villi (villous atrophy)
2. Increased mitotic activity in the crypt zone
3. Increase in the population of intra-epithelial lymphocytes

201 1. Giant rugal hypertrophy of the stomach
2. Gastric cancer
3. Whipple's disease
4. Regional ileitis
5. Ulcerative colitis
6. Tropical and non-tropical sprue syndromes

202 The commonest cause of intestinal infarction is a vascular block in the intestinal blood vessels caused by atheroma, thrombosis or an embolus. Blockage of the superior mesenteric artery at its origin causes infarction of the whole of the small bowel except for the duodenum, and the caecum and ascending and transverse colon.

203 The gut is said to be strangulated when its blood supply is severely impaired by external pressure as in a hernia. First the venous return is compromised because veins are more easily compressed than arteries but as congestion develops so the arterial supply is reduced. Other causes of strangulation include fibrous bands and adhesions, intussusception and volvulus.

204 The oral administration of enteric coated potassium chloride or hydrochlorthiazide tablets. How these compounds cause ulceration is unclear. At first small and punched out, the ulcers gradually enlarge circumferentially to produce annular lesions.

205   1. Serpiginous, discontinuous mucosal ulceration, at first superficial but later involving all layers of the gut except for the serosa
      2. Stricture formation, short or long, single or multiple. The thickening of the bowel at the site of a stricture gives rise to the term, 'hosepipe' stricture
      3. In approximately one-quarter of cases the mucosa has a 'cobblestone' appearance. This is due to oedema of the surviving mucosa between the linear ulcers.
      4. 'Skip' lesions. In some patients a number of separate lesions may be present with apparently normal bowel in between.

206   1. In the majority of cases a sarcoid or tuberculoid type of lesion is found in the affected bowel and local lymph nodes. The absence of caseation distinguishes the condition from tuberculosis.
      2. Clefts or fissures lined by granulation tissue containing both epithelioid and giant cells penetrate deeply into the bowel wall.
      3. Lymphocytes and plasmacytes may be found diffusely scattered or in focal aggregates some with germinal centres, throughout all layers of affected bowel.
      4. Diffuse oedema is present in all layers of the bowel.
      5. Fibrosis

207   Any part. However, when Crohn described the condition in 1922 he considered it to be a chronic inflammatory disease affecting only the terminal ileum. Since 1960 it has gradually been appreciated that the disease can affect any part of the gastrointestinal tract including the mouth and anus and that both the skin and joints may be involved.

208   This condition is inherited through an autosomal gene. Bluish, ill-defined spots develop in the lips and buccal mucosa and freckles appear in the circumoral skin. Sessile or pedunculated polyps develop, chiefly in the jejunum and occasionally in the stomach and colon. Microscopic examination of the polyps shows them to be due to proliferated muscularis mucosae and the overlying epithelium is normal.

209   1. The site of the lesion. Ulcerative colitis

involves only the rectum and colon although in severe disease the terminal ileum may be affected producing so-called 'back-wash' ileitis. In contrast, Crohn's disease may affect any part of the gastrointestinal tract.

2. Extent of mural involvement. Ulcerative colitis is essentially a mucosal disease. Ulcers with undermined edges develop and the surviving mucosa becomes oedematous and inflamed. Tags of such mucosa are described as pseudopolyps. In contrast Crohn's disease involves all layers of the bowel causing typical 'hose-pipe' strictures. Adhesions between the loops or between an involved loop and the abdominal parietes may result in an internal or external fistula.

3. Histological appearances. In ulcerative proctocolitis prior to the development of ulceration, 'crypt' abscesses develop, the mucosal glands becoming filled with pus cells. In Crohn's disease non-caseating granulomata develop in both the wall of the gut and the adjacent lymph nodes. The deep fissures which develop in this disease can be seen with the naked eye and the oedema of the intervening mucosa produces the typical 'cobblestone' appearance.

4. Malignant change. Only in ulcerative colitis is malignancy likely to develop. The frequently of this complication is related to the extent and duration of the disease.

210 1. In the former the polyps predominantly occur in the small intestine whereas in the latter polyps are only present in the colon and rectum.
2. Familial polyposis is not associated with mucocutaneous pigmentation.
3. Jejunal and ileal polyps never become malignant whereas the colonic polyps associated with familial polyposis inevitably do after some years, multiple malignancies being common.

211 All primary tumours of the small gut are rare. They include:
1. carcinoid tumours, also known as apudomata or argentaffinomata
2. lymphomata which may be associated with gluten-induced enteropathy when they are frequently multiple
3. adenocarcinomata which may cause bleeding, intussusception or intestinal obstruction

212 A carcinoid tumour arises from the APUD (Amine Precursor Uptake and Decarboxylation) cells of the gastrointestinal tract. Such tumours are also known as argentaffinomata or enterochromaffin cell tumours because of their silver-staining properties. The cells of this system by decarboxylating the precursors produce biological active amines such as 5-hydroxytryptamine (5-HT).

The commonest site of origin of these tumours is in the appendix where they may cause obstructive appendicitis. From this site they usually metastasise late and do not produce hormonal effects presumably because the 5-HT is detoxified in the liver before it enters the systemic from the portal blood. The second commonest site of origin is the lower ileum. In this site they may cause simple mechanical obstruction. The tumours become hormonally active and the carcinoid syndrome develops when secondaries occur in the liver and the 5-HT spills into the general circulation. The chief features of this syndrome are:
1. patchy flushing of the face which may be markedly and persistently cyanosed
2. intermittent diarrhoea
3. signs of tricuspid and pulmonary stenosis or incompetence due to thickening of the valve cusps, atrial wall and ventricular endocardium.

The diagnosis of an active tumour is confirmed by finding excessive quantities of 5-hydroxyindole acetic acid, a breakdown product of 5-hydroxytryptamine, in the urine.

213 1. Perforation leading to general peritonitis, an appendix abscess or a localised abscess anywhere in the peritoneal cavity. An appendix abscess, once established, may slowly resolve or alternatively progress and 'point' i.e. perforate the abdominal wall or into another viscus producing a fistula.
2. Portal pyaemia
3. Mucocoele. This condition usually follows acute inflammation. The appendix is distended with mucus and the wall is pale and attenuated. Rupture of a mucocoele may lead to the development of pseudomyxoma peritonei which is frequently complicated by small bowel obstructions.

214 The term 'necrotising enterocolitis' was originally

coined to describe a condition in which varying degrees of necrosis of the intestinal mucosa occurred, leading to such severe diarrhoea that death from hypovolaemic shock nearly always occurred. The following causes have been recognised:
1. ischaemia of the gut with or without secondary infection by intestinal flora normally present there, e.g. anaerobic clostridia
2. severe staphylococcal and viral infections not associated with ischaemia
3. overgrowth of exotoxin-producing staphylococci following antibiotic therapy in patients undergoing partial gastrectomy
4. prematurity followed by a bacterial or viral infection of the gut.

215 Hirschsprung's disease is a congenital condition commoner in boys than girls, affecting the terminal large bowel. The parasympathetic ganglia are absent from Auerbach's and Meissner's plexuses and there is an increase in non-myelinated nerve fibres in the submucosa and between the circular and longitudinal muscle coats. This neurological abnormality causes uncoordinated muscular contraction of the affected region of the bowel leading to physiological intestinal obstruction. The disease is recognised within a few days of birth in 75 per cent of affected babies and in the remainder within three months. Most commonly the abnormality extends proximally from the ano-rectal junction for several centimetres but in 10 per cent of patients, the whole of the large bowel and even the small bowel may be affected.

216 Diverticular disease of the colon is defined as a condition in which multiple diverticula, associated with thickening of both the taenia coli and the circular muscle of the colon occur. In simple diverticulosis there is no inflammation whereas an outstanding feature of diverticulitis is the presence of inflammatory changes particularly involving the pericolic and mesenteric fat.

The reason for superadded inflammation to the diverticula is, as in the case of appendicitis, not completely understood but is probably the result of poor drainage or faecolith formation in the diverticula. No specific organism is incriminated.

217 Diverticular disease most commonly occurs in people who eat a low roughage rather than a bulky vegetable diet. Rats fed on a low residue diet develop diverticula. It is believed that prior to the appearance of the diverticula themselves, changes occur in the muscular wall of the gut which lead to a sustained intraluminal pressure in the colon. This leads to pulsion diverticula as the mucosa is thrust through the bowel wall where it is weakest, i.e. where the blood vessels penetrate the muscular coats.

218 1. Diverticulitis. Inflammation begins at the apex of the diverticula and having penetrated the mucosa, may spread in the muscle layers producing widespread changes which later, after resolving, may cause longitudinal scarring and stricture formation. Alternatively, the severity of the infection may be such that perforation of the colon occurs leading either to a pericolic abscess or, in rare cases, a faecal peritonitis.
2. Haemorrhage. Clinically unrecognisable quantities of blood may be lost from inflamed diverticula but on rare occasions the involvement of a larger colonic artery may lead to a sudden massive haemorrhage.
3. Intestinal obstruction. Repeated attacks of inflammation followed by resolution can lead to a stricture.
4. Fistulae. Fistulae associated with diverticulitis may be external or internal, most frequently the latter. Although almost any hollow organ may be involved the commonest internal fistula is that between the colon and bladder.

219 'Back-wash' ileitis describes the changes in the terminal ileum which occur in patients suffering from chronic total colitis. The villi and crypts are destroyed and the ileal mucosa becomes reddened, granular and ulcerated. It is possibly due to reflux of the caecal contents through an incompetent ileocaecal valve or it may be merely an extension of the inflammatory process in the colon.

220 The term 'polyp' is devoid of pathological significance. It merely indicates the presence of a circumscribed tumour which projects from the mucous membrane. A polyp may be sessile or,

possessing a stalk of variable length, pedunculated. There are four main histological types:
1. neoplastic (adenomatous or malignant)
2. hamartomatous
3. inflammatory
4. unclassified

221 The WHO classify adenomatous polyps or adenomata as:
1. tubular adenomata
2. villous adenomata
3. tubulo-villous adenomata which are a mixture of the above

Most adenomata are mixed.

222 1. Familial polyposis
2. Ulcerative colitis
3. Schistosomiasis
4. Pre-existing adenomata

223 Adenomata of the large bowel are liable to malignant change. Villous adenomata are considered to be at greater risk than tubular adenomata. Assessment of malignancy in an adenoma may be difficult and depends on dysplastic cellular changes. No matter how dysplastic the cells, metastases cannot occur so long as the growth has not breached the muscularis mucosae since no lymphatics are present in the lamina propria to permit dissemination of tumour cell emboli.

224 Three-quarters of all large bowel cancers arise in the sigmoid colon or rectum. They are frequently multiple and may be associated with adenomata from which most carcinomata are considered to arise. Most of the growths are ulcerating with rolled edges and many become annular to produce a tight stricture. Some are protuberant and have a villous appearance suggesting origin from a villous adenoma. Others are 'colloid' cancers, i.e. produce copious mucin. Colorectal carcinomata, unlike gastric, tend to be small and circumscribed and rarely infiltrate diffusely as in the case of linitis plastica.

Microscopically, most are well-differentiated adenocarcinomata with a marked glandular pattern and are of an average grade of malignancy. Ten per cent are mucinous, with mucin in cellular vacuoles or lying between cells. Undifferentiated or anaplastic carcinomata are rare.

225 Duke's classification of colorectal cancers defines the degree of spread of a tumour. It is one guide to prognosis although other factors such as the degree of histological dedifferentiation should also be taken into account.

Duke's A. The tumour has neither spread beyond the muscularis propria nor spread by the lymphatics.

Duke's B. The tumour has spread through the muscularis propria into the pericolic or perirectal tissues although no lymphatic involvement is present.

Duke's C. The tumour is associated with lymphatic metastases irrespective of the degree of direct spread. Cure is impossible and only one-third of patients in this group survive for more than five years.

226 A raised carcinoembryonic antigen (CEA) level in the blood was initially considered to be associated only with carcinoma of the colon. This has now been disproved and it has been shown that CEA may be raised in other tumours, in cirrhosis of the liver and in viral hepatitis. However, a rapid rise in the CEA following the removal of colorecral cancer indicates recurrent tumour with rapid deterioration of the patient.

LIVER & GALL BLADDER

227 This rare condition is due to obstruction of the hepatic vein, either by compression by tumour from without or by a thrombus or a large tumour embolism within. Endophlebitis with thrombosis of the hepatic vein is the commonest cause but the aetiology is unknown. Acute hepatic sinusoidal dilatation and massive ascites result from this.

228 1. Protozoa
   a. Amoebae causing abscesses secondary to amoebic dysentery
   b. Malaria parasites
   c. Leishmania causing kala-azar (visceral leishmaniasis)
2. Metazoa
   a. Schistosomiasis
   b. *Echinococcus granulosus* (hydatid disease)
   c. Liver flukes (clonorchis and fasciola)
   d. Ascaris. The round worm which obstructs the common bile duct

229 Chronic persistent hepatitis is a mild disease. Clinically there are vague symptoms of malaise, abdominal pain, slightly enlarged liver and slight biochemical changes in the blood. Portal tracts have a little lymphoid cell infiltrate and there is minimal, if any, hepatocellular damage. Cirrhosis does not occur unless the condition becomes chronic active hepatitis which happens occasionally.

Chronic active hepatitis is a more severe condition, in many cases starting as acute HB viral hepatitis. Symptoms are as above but with signs of liver failure and splenomegaly. In addition there are skin rashes, serous effusions, glomerular lesions causing proteinuria and conditions indicating an auto-immune state, e.g. chronic thyroiditis. Histologically, degeneration of liver cells is prominent, particularly 'piecemeal necrosis' where hepatocytes adjacent to fibrosis are being destroyed. Cirrhosis is a common sequel.

Both types of chronic hepatitis are thought to be the outcome of acute viral hepatitis infection.

230 Cirrhosis consists of nodularity of the whole liver caused by a process of destruction and regeneration of the parenchyma with the formation of bands of collagenous fibrous tissue which separate the nodules. The regenerated nodules have lost the normal hepatic architecture, hepatocytes may show fatty vacuolation (indicating continuing toxic onslaught), there is a variable lymphoid cell infiltrate in portal tracts and the collagen bands, and hepatocellular jaundice may be present. The liver may be enlarged or of normal size but it usually becomes small in time. The classification of the various forms of cirrhosis for practical purposes is by aetiology rather than liver morphology, such as the size of the nodules.

231 1. Scattered hepatocytes may die: apoptosis
2. Focal necrosis, this occurs in portal pyaemia and acute viral or drug-induced hepatitis. Such foci are not situated it any particular part of the liver lobules.
3. Zonal necrosis:
   a. periportal necrosis occurs in phosphorus poisoning
   b. central zonal (centrilobular) necrosis occurs in anaemia, chronic venous congestion and alcoholic poisoning
   c. midzone necrosis occurs in yellow fever

4. Massive hepatic necrosis (acute yellow atrophy) may be caused by the hepatitis virus or exposure to hepatotoxic drugs such as carbon tetrachloride.

232
1. Alcoholic
2. Post-viral
3. Biliary cirrhosis, of unknown aetiology or due to mechanical obstruction of the larger biliary passages
4. Cryptogenic

233 Primary biliary cirrhosis is uncommon and its aetiology is unknown. It is eight times commoner in women. The onset is insidious with ill health and mild jaundice at first. The liver is enlarged and serum cholesterol is increased thus predisposing to subcutaneous xanthelasmata. Malabsorption occurs in chronic cases. The jaundice is obstructive.

Histologically, the intrahepatic bile ducts are destroyed by non-suppurative inflammation. Lymphocytes and plasma cells are present in large numbers round the smaller bile ducts where sarcoid-like granulomata develop in a third of cases. The inflammation extends periportally to some extent destroying adjacent hepatocytes, and the portal tracts eventually become fibrosed which causes cholestasis. Continuing hepatocyte destruction with regeneration and fibrosis results in a micronodular cirrhosis.

234 In sclerosing cholangitis the extrahepatic and occasionally the larger intrahepatic biliary ducts become progressively obliterated by fibrosis. This eventually leads to biliary cirrhosis and portal hypertension. The condition is usually secondary to acute infective cholangitis caused by stones in the biliary tree but it is occasionally associated with chronic ulcerative colitis and retroperitoneal fibrosis.

235 Primary biliary cirrhosis is not infrequently associated with scleroderma, rheumatoid arthritis and Sjögren's syndrome. These associations together with marked lymphoid cell infiltrate in the liver suggest alterations in the immune mechanism. This is borne out by:
1. elevation of serum gamma globulins, particularly the IgM fraction

2. the presence of mitochondrial antibodies
   3. a reduction in T-cell responsiveness in about half the patients

236 1. Jaundice: the severity reflects the degree of hepatocellular damage
   2. Peripheral oedema due to diminished production of albumin
   3. Endocrine disturbances, notably testicular atrophy and gynaecomastia in the male due to failure of the liver to inactivate oestrogens
   4. Bleeding tendency due to diminished production of prothrombin, fibrinogen and Factors V, VII, IX and X

237 1. Malignant.
   a. The most common are secondary carcinomata from almost any primary, usually of alimentary, pulmonary or breast origin
   b. Primary malignant tumours of liver
      (i) Hepatocellular carcinomata, a complication of cirrhosis
      (ii) Cholangiocarcinomata, not related to cirrhosis but associated with liver fluke infestation and hence commoner in the Far East
   2. Benign are uncommon
   a. Liver cell adenomata
   b. Bile duct adenomata
   c. Haemangiomata, usually cavernous and dark purple; they may be mistaken for secondary melanomata

238 Ninety per cent of all cases of acute cholecystitis are associated with gall stones. In the early stages the gall bladder is distended, the serosal surface is congested and the wall thickened and oedematous. Microscopically gross vascular dilatation is present together with a diffuse scattering of mononuclear and polymorphonuclear leucocytes. In the early stages bacteria are not necessarily seen.

If the outlet of the gall bladder is blocked, either by severe oedema or the presence of a stone, the inflammatory process increases in severity and becomes haemorrhagic or suppurative. Abscesses form in the wall and gangrene may occur. When the lumen is filled with pus the condition is known as an empyema of the gall bladder. Gangrene leads to perforation and the development of biliary peritonitis, but less severe disease may undergo resolution leaving a fibrosed, thick-walled, shrunken organ. Occasionally adherence to the duodenum leads to an internal fistula between it and the gall bladder.

239   1. A high calorie diet
2. Hyperglycaemia
3. A high cholesterol diet
4. A decreased conversion of cholesterol to bile acids in the liver
5. Oestrogenic or progestational hormones
6. A reduced chenodeoxycholic/cholic acid ratio

240   This is not fully understood except in the case of pure pigment stones which result from chronic haemolysis. Most stones are mixed and the following are predisposing factors:
1. the composition of the bile.
   a. Supersaturation with cholesterol
   b. The detergent effect of bile acids which keeps cholesterol in solution.
   Thus the ratio of a. to b. is important
2. physico-chemical changes in the mucus secreted by the gall bladder mucosa
3. infection may be responsible for initiating stone formation or may potentiate the preceding

241   1. Pure, otherwise known as metabolic stones, consisting chiefly of cholesterol, calcium carbonate or bile pigment. Cholesterol and carbonate stones are commonly solitary whereas pigment stones are always multiple.
2. Mixed, otherwise known as infective stones. These consist of layers of bile pigments and cholesterol both containing an admixture of calcium salts and organic material. They are always multiple and faceted due to their growth while the stones are in apposition.

242   Gall stone ileus is the term applied to intestinal obstruction due to a large gall stone impacting in the lumen of the lower ileum. The gall stone enters the duodenum by causing pressure atrophy of the gall bladder and adjacent duodenal walls to produce a cholecyst-duodenal fistula. There is usually a history of previous attacks of acute cholecystitis.

243 Acute pancreatitis is the result of destruction of the gland by activated pancreatic enzymes, especially phospholipidase A, chymotrypsin, kallikrein and elastase. Trypsin probably functions as an enzyme activator rather than destroying pancreatic tissue. Lipase participates in extra-pancreatic fat necrosis. How the proenzymes become activated within the pancreas is unknown but the following suggestions have been made:
1. in patients suffering from cholelithiasis stones temporarily impacted in the ampulla of Vater might cause the reflux of bile into the pancreatic duct under increased pressure, alternatively such a stone might allow the reflux of duodenal contents into the duct. In a high proportion of patients suffering from gall stone pancreatitis stones can be found in the stools if these are sieved immediately after an attack.
2. in both chronic alcoholism and hypercalcaemia it is thought that sustained pancreatic hypersecretion is responsible for the development of pancreatitis. The hypothesis is that with sustained hypersecretion there is precipitation of mucoprotein and calcium carbonate which causes plugging of the smaller pancreatic ducts and thus localised areas of pancreatic necrosis.

244 Acute pancreatitis is a disease of variable severity, not all parts of the gland being equally affected. The disease is divided into three degrees of severity:
1. oedematous pancreatitis, in which the gland is focally or diffusely oedematous and a slight lymphoid cell infiltration is present
2. haemorrhagic pancreatitis, in which there is marked parenchymal destruction together with interstitial and peripancreatic haemorrhage accompanied by extensive leucocytic (mainly polymorph) infiltration. Necrosis of the peripancreatic fat occurs. Vasculitis with thrombi in venules is characteristic
3. gangrenous pancreatitis, in which the gland becomes a necrotic amorphous mass

245 1. Gall stones
2. Chronic alcoholism
3. A raised serum calcium

4. Hyperlipidaemia, especially Types I and V
5. Viral infections; mumps, Coxsackie and Echo viruses
6. Certain drugs among which are included azathioprine, oestrogens and sulphonamides

246 This disease is associated with atrophy and fibrosis, sometimes with calcification of the gland. The parenchyma is markedly reduced therefore causing a reduction of exocrine secretions and hence steatorrhoea. In severe cases the islet cell tissue is also destroyed, causing diabetes. The cellular infiltrate in the diseased gland consists mainly of lymphocytes and plasma cells.

247 1. Death; in the early stages this may be due to hypovolaemic shock and in the later stages to infection
2. Pseudocyst formation; these arise from the rupture of pancreatic ducts with leakage of active enzymes beyond the boundaries of the pancreas. Commonly unilocular pseudo-pancreatic cysts fill the lesser sac and then may extend. They have no epithelial lining
3. Abscess formation; when bacterial infection occurs in necrotic pancreatic tissue an abscess develops which may eventually spread to any site in the peritoneal cavity

248 Carcinoma of the pancreas is an adenocarcinoma which is usually well-differentiated. It presents insidiously. Two major symptoms may lead to clinical suspicion; the development of constant lower thoracic back pain probably caused by extra-pancreatic spread and secondly, painless progressive jaundice possibly associated with a palpable enlarged gall bladder due to pressure on the common bile duct. Phlebitis migrans is associated with this tumour.

NERVOUS SYSTEM

249 1. Bleeding. The classic example of this is tearing of the middle meningeal artery or vein when the temporal bone is fractured, giving rise to an extradural haemorrhage. Subdural, sub-arachnoid and intracerebral haemorrhages may also occur.
2. Infection. Compound fractures of the skull or

fractures involving the air sinuses may be complicated by infection of the cranium, the subdural or subarachnoid spaces or the brain itself.

3. Aerocoele (pneumatocoele cranii—air under the scalp). An aerocoele develops when bone forming the wall of a paranasal sinus is fractured. If the meninges are torn an aerocoele can rupture into a ventricle.
4. Leakage of cerebrospinal fluid. Cerebrospinal rhinorrhoea may follow a fracture of the frontal, ethmoidal or sphenoidal sinuses whereas a fracture of the temporal bone may be followed by otorrhoea. Infection may supervene in each case.
5. Damage to cranial nerves. Any cranial nerve may be injured if the fracture line involves a foramen. The olfactory nerves are particularly susceptible because of their relatively slender structure.
6. Brain lacerations.
7. Epilepsy. Damage to the cerebral cortex followed by gliosis may result in post-traumatic focal epilepsy.

250 According to the severity of the injury the following may occur:
1. concussion. Unconsciousness immediately following a head injury only occurs if the head moves in response to a blow, thus causing sudden acceleration or deceleration of the brain within the rigid cranium. The opportunity to examine the brain when only transient unconsciousness has occurred is rare but the following pathological changes have been described:
   a. red cells and plasma in the circumvascular (Virchow-Robin) spaces which is a non-specific reaction
   b. axonal 'retraction bulbs', formed from beads of axoplasm which escape after an axon is severed
   c. microglial scars
2. contusion. A contusion is a cluster of more or less confluent petechial haemorrhages associated with variable degrees of necrosis. In a deceleration injury a large contusion may develop at a site diametrically opposite to the point of impact, the so-called 'contrecoup' injury. Small contusions may heal completely

whereas larger ones may be followed by atrophy of the cortex and yellow staining of the pia mater. Microscopic examination reveals gliosis in the affected area and the presence of haemosiderin-containing macrophages, surrounded by a zone of astrocytosis.
3. laceration. This is tearing of cortical surface and overlying pia-arachnoid. Lacerations of the brain are associated with subarachnoid or subdural haemorrhage or gross interstitial haemorrhage.

251 Wallerian degeneration describes the changes which occur when a nerve fibre is separated from its nerve cell.

Within 12 hours fragmentation of the axon can be observed, after which the myelin and the axon form ovoid bodies surrounded by proliferating Schwann cells.

The rate of degeneration is determined by:
1. myelination; heavily myelinated fibres degenerate more rapidly than the unmyelinated
2. function; sensory fibres degenerate faster than motor nerves.

With axonal and myelin degeneration, macrophages, fibroblasts and perineural cells form continuous columns, known as von Bungner's bands. This is the architectural scaffold within which the regenerating axon grows.

At the same time that these changes are taking place distal to the point of section, central chromatolysis occurs in the perikaryon of the parent nerve cell body. This leaves the nerve cell with a thin peripheral rind of Nissl substance. Such changes are not degenerative but merely a response of the nerve cell prior to regenerative activity.

252 1. Lead. Chronic lead poisoning causes dementia probably due to cerebral ischaemia produced by proliferation of the endothelium of the small blood vessels.
2. Mercury. Chronic mercury poisoning causes widespread degeneration in the central nervous system especially in the granular layer of the cerebellar cortex and calcarine area of the cerebral cortex. The classic symptoms of mercury poisoning in the adult are profuse salivation, a coarse tremor and emotional instability. In young children it produces pink disease.

3. **Manganese.** Chronic manganese poisoning causes loss of neurones in the cerebral cortex, basal ganglia and cerebellum. The result is extra-pyramidal rigidity and a coarse tremor.
4. **Tin.** This metal is a rare cause of neurological disturbance but the ingestion of organic compounds of this metal causes cerebral oedema.

253 A dysraphic malformation is a congenital abnormality in which the neural tube fails to fuse. Four varieties are recognised:
1. craniorachischis in which the whole neural tube remains open
2. anencephaly when the neural groove of the brain fails to close
3. encephalocoele and meningocoele when failure of closure is limited to the rostral part of the neural tube
4. spina bifida when the defect is limited to the lumbar segments

254 1. Spina bifida occulta. In this condition the vertebral arches of the lumbar region fail to fuse. There is no defect in the spinal cord or roots; the meninges are intact but the site of the defect may be marked in the skin by a dimple, hairy patch or pigmented area.
2. Spina bifida cystica. This may present as:
   a. a meningocoele when a cystic protrusion of the meninges is present beneath the skin but the cord and roots are normal
   b. a myelomeningocoele when the skin over the cyst is absent and the meninges are exposed or even deficient. The arrangement of the cord and nerves is very variable and absence of normal development leads to defective function of the sphincters and paralysis of the lower limbs. A high incidence of hydrocephalus and the Arnold-Chiari malformation are associated with this condition. Infection of the central nervous system eventually occurs if untreated.

255 Down's syndrome is caused by the failure of chromosome 21 to separate during oogenesis with the result that three of these chromosomes are present in a fertilized ovum. Thus the chromosomal composition of a typical Down's baby is 47,XX +21 or 47,XY, +21, this formula indicating the

presence of a male or female with an additional 21 chromosome, a genotype known as trisomy 21. This type of Down's syndrome is commonest in women who bear children towards the end of their reproductive life.

A rarer form of Down's syndrome, not related to maternal age, is associated with 46 chromosomes. One of these is large and is composed of 21 attached to 15, constituting a translocation. Thus the normal complement of chromosomes is present and the trisomy is latent.

256 All are rare. They include:
1. the leucodystrophies
2. the neuronal lipidoses: amaurotic familial idiocy and Niemann-Pick and Gaucher's diseases
3. Phenylketonuria

257 1. Peroneal muscular atrophy (Charcot-Marie-Tooth disease).
2. Friedreich's ataxia.
3. Infantile progressive spinal muscular atrophy (Werdnig-Hoffmann disease).

258 The former is a specific form of degeneration of the central nervous system inherited as a Mendelian dominant and is associated with choreoathetosis and mental deterioration, whereas the latter is a manifestation of acute rheumatic fever in which no specific histological changes in the central nervous system are found.

259 They most commonly develop alongside the superior sagittal sinus following the rupture, due to trauma, of veins in their passage between the arachnoid and dura mater. The bleeding may be so rapid that sudden compression of the underlying brain is produced together with a cerebellar pressure cone followed by death. Alternatively a slow increase in intracranial pressure may occur caused by the liquefaction of a clot and the absorption of fluid into it. The symptoms and signs of the latter are those of an expanding intracranial lesion, usually with marked lateralising signs.

260 The commonest sites for brain haemorrhage are:
1. the lentiform nucleus, due to bleeding from the lenticulostriate branch of the middle cerebral artery

2. the pons
3. the white matter of the cerebelllum

The major predisposing factors are:
1. hypertension causing rupture of an atherosclerotic vessel or a microaneurysm
2. A pre-existing brain lesion, e.g. a primary or secondary neoplasm or a septic focus

Death usually occurs following brain haemorrhage due to extension of the haematoma in the cortex or rupture into a ventricle.

261 1. Congenital defects in the media leading to the development of 'berry' aneurysms. Although structural weakness in the media is common the development of an aneurysm is rare. This type of aneurysm most frequently occurs in the middle cerebral artery either at its origin or where it branches.
2. Atherosclerosis.
3. Hypertension.
4. Mycotic, arising in patients suffering from subacute bacterial endocarditis.

262 The middle cerebral, in particular the lenticulostriate branch which supplies that part of the internal capsule which is traversed by the axons of the motor cells in the precentral gyrus as they pass to the cord. Thrombosis of this artery destroys the axons and myelin sheaths in the affected part of the internal capsule resulting in a contralateral hemiplegia. Sensation is preserved because the afferent fibres are situated further back in the internal capsule.

263 Spontaneous thrombosis of the superior longitudinal venous sinus of the brain. It occurs in poorly nourished children who develop an acute infection and in cachetic adults suffering from malignant disease or an infective fever, such as malaria. If the obstruction is complete, intense engorgement of the superficial veins of the brain occurs. This frequently leads to haemorrhagic infarction of the parasagittal areas of the cerebral hemispheres. Thrombosis in the straight sinus causes similar changes in the walls of the third ventricle.

264 The appearance of a cerebral infarct depends upon its age and the associated vascular changes.
  A fresh infarct appears as a swollen area usually ovoid in shape which is softer than the

surrounding brain tissue. If necrosis of the vessel walls in the area of the infarct has occurred the infarct is red because of the extravasation of blood from the damaged vessels whereas if the vessels remain intact a pale infarct is produced which, when fresh, may be difficult to distinguish from the normal brain tissue. Within a few weeks the central part of all infarcts liquefies to produce a yellow, gelatinous material which later becomes fluid.

Microscopically, at an early stage, ischaemic necrosis of the neurones occurs. This is followed by the ingress of phagocytes which take up lipid globules derived from myelin degeneration, and haemosiderin from extravasated degenerate erythrocytes. At the periphery, capillary and glial cell proliferation occurs, eventually producing encapsulation.

265 Pachymeningitis is an inflammatory lesion of the dura and leptomeningitis an inflammation of the pia and arachnoid.

Pachymeningitis is rarer than leptomeningitis and is usually caused by the direct spread of infection from the bones of the skull, e.g. following a compound fracture or suppurative otitis media whereas leptomeningitis is caused by organisms carried to the meninges via the blood stream.

266 Gross changes:
1. the dura mater is thickened
2. there may be unilateral or bilateral chronic subdural haematoma
3. the arachnoid mater is thickened and opaque
4. the gyri are atrophied and, in consequence, the sulci are broadened and contain an excess of cerebrospinal fluid
5. the ventricles are enlarged because of cerebral atrophy
6. granular ependymitis occurs

Microscopic changes:
1. the cellularity of the grey matter is increased due to an excess of neuroglial cells
2. the small blood vessels are surrounded by cuffs of lymphocytes and plasma cells
3. the astrocytes are enlarged and branched and are described as 'spider' cells
4. the microglial cells increase in number and may contain iron granules
5. there is neuronal loss

6. gliosis may be present in the subjacent white matter

267
1. Penetrating injuries of the brain
2. Direct spread of infection from neighbouring septic foci, for example:
   a. temporal lobe abscess following otitis media
   b. cerebellar abscess following mastoiditis
   c. frontal lobe abscess following frontal, ethmoidal or sphenoidal infection
3. Haematogenous infection from:
   a. the lungs, e.g. in bronchiectasis
   b. the heart in infective endocarditis

268 The cytomegalovirus is a herpes virus chiefly affecting newborn babies via the transplacental route. Changes develop in many tissues, the colonised cells becoming greatly enlarged due to distension of the nucleus by inclusion bodies which may also be intracytoplasmic. In infants, death is the result of an encephalitis and children who survive may be mentally retarded or develop hydrocephalus. In adults, many of whom have serological evidence of infection, only a mild or subclinical disease mimicking infectious mononucleosis may occur. This virus is a cause of opportunistic infection in individuals of all ages who are immunodeficient.

269 A disease in which the myelin sheaths of the nerve fibres disappear. This may be a primary phenomenon when, despite the destruction of the myelin sheath, the axon remains at least for a time intact, or it may be secondary in which case the axon is first destroyed with the ensuing disappearance of the myelin.

Primary demyelination follows many viral infections such as measles, varicella, rubella and mumps. A similar condition, post-vaccinial encephalomyelopathy, follows vaccination against smallpox.

Other than infective causes the most important demyelinating disease is multiple sclerosis. The aetiology of this condition remains obscure, laboratory investigation being hindered by the absence of a comparable disease in animals.

270 The commonest pathological change is the development of areas of demyelination, described as plaques. These occur in any part of the central

nervous system but are particularly common in the white matter surrounding the lateral ventricles and in the optic nerves. Plaques of recent origin are yellow or pink in colour and soft in consistency whereas older plaques are grey and firm.

Histology frequently shows the presence of a venule in or near the centre of a recent plaque surrounded by macrophages filled with the lipid breakdown products of myelin. In older lesions the macrophages are surrounded by lymphocytes.

Special stains are required to show the loss of myelin and the proliferation of glial fibres in the plaques.

271 The Lewy body. This is particularly common in the pigmented cells of the substantia nigra and corpora cerulea. These acidophil bodies may be so large that the cell containing them becomes unrecognisable.

272   1. Primary tumours:
   a. neuronal tend to occur in childhood and are malignant; neuroblastoma, medulloblastoma and retinoblastoma
   b. neuroglial are all malignant but variably so
       (i) gliomata are better differentiated histologically and are slower growing. They are named after the cell of origin and include astrocytoma; oligodendroglioma; ependymoma.
       (ii) anaplastic gliomata e.g. glioblastoma multiforme are most malignant
   c. meningioma, commonly benign
   d. nerve sheath and nerve root tumours, all benign
       (i) schwannoma (neurilemmoma, acoustic neuroma)
       (ii) traumatic neuroma
       (iii) neurofibroma may become malignant when multiple (von Recklinghausen's disease)
   e. Uncommon tumours and cysts
       (i) angioma, a developmental malformation
       (ii) haemangioblastoma is malignant
       (iii) epidermoid cyst
       (iv) teratoma, malignant or benign (dermoid cyst)
       (v) craniopharyngioma (supracellar cyst), benign
   2. Secondary tumours are common and may be

the first indication of malignant disease in almost any other part of the body.

273 Tumours derived from the Schwann cells may arise along the course of any cranial or spinal nerve. The commonest intracranial site of origin is from the vestibulocochlear nerve, the tumour arising just outside the internal acoustic meatus.

Normally solid, Schwann cell tumours may undergo central liquefactive necrosis. Microscopically they consist of interlacing bands of spindle cells, the nuclei of adjacent cells appearing to be aligned in parallel columns producing 'palisading'.

274 A meningioma is a tumour developing from the specialised arachnoid cells of the villi which project into the dural sinuses. It most commonly arises in the region of the superior sagittal sinus but may occur in the spinal canal where it arises from the dura over the lateral aspect of the spinal cord, or from the arachnoid tissue on the dural reflections over the spinal roots.

Meningiomata grow slowly producing smooth or nodular, friable, encapsulated white tumours with erosion of overlying bone. They have a variable microscopic appearance. The commonest variety, the syncytial type is composed of poorly defined polygonal cells. Less common is the transitional type composed of nests of cells arranged concentrically in whorls which calcify to form gritty psammoma bodies.

URINARY SYSTEM

275 Infantile and adult, both are inherited. The former is due to an autosomal recessive and the latter an autosomal dominant gene. In the infantile type, which is rare, the kidneys are enlarged and the renal tissue is so completely replaced by cysts developing from the proximal convoluted tubules that death occurs in infancy. The adult type is fairly common and usually presents between 20 to 40 years of age with hypertension or uraemia. Cysts of varying size bulge from the surface of the enlarged kidneys and any normal tissue present undergoes pressure atrophy.

276 Carbon tetrachloride, trilene, diethylene glycol, carbolic acid, organic mercurials and metallic mercury, uranium, arsenic and chromium.

277   1. Randall's theory.
Randall suggested that crystalloid precipitation commences in the distal collecting tubules deep to the urothelium covering the pyramids. Once the microscopic concretion is large enough the urothelium overlying it ulcerates and then it either falls free into the renal pelvis to be passed or it grows *in situ* to macroscopic proportions.
2. Carr's theory.
Carr suggests that the initial crystalline deposit occurs in the lymphatics surrounding the base of a pyramid when these are either overloaded with crystalline material or obstructed by inflammatory change.

278   1. Calcium oxalate. These are nodular or spiculated, frequently black in colour, due to a covering of altered blood.
2. Phosphate stones. Off-white or grey in colour, this type of stone may grow to fill the pelvis and calyces forming a 'stag-horn' calculus.
3. Uric acid stones, yellowish brown, hard and smooth.
4. Cystine stones, yellowish, soft and waxy and frequently multiple.

279   1. Hypercalciuria. Idiopathic or secondary to other conditions such as hyperparathyroidism, myelomatosis, renal acidosis, sarcoidosis or recumbency.
2. Hyperuricaemia from any cause, e.g. gout, leukaemia, polycythaemia.
3. Inborn errors or metabolism leading to hyperoxaluria, cystinuria and xanthinuria.
4. Mechanical factors causing the stagnation of urine, e.g. medullary sponge kidney.
5. Infection by urea-splitting organisms such as B. proteus which produce ammonia and thus an alkaline urine. This causes the formation of stones composed of ammonium magnesium phosphate.

280   1. Impaction anywhere between the pelvi-ureteric junction and the distal end of the ureter may lead to loss of renal function.
2. Infection, most commonly by E. coli and other enteric bacteria.
3. Squamous metaplasia of the urothelium lining the renal pelvis which may finally lead to the development of a squamous carcinoma at this site.

281 Renal tuberculosis arises by haematogenous spread of *Mycobacterium tuberculosis* from a focus elsewhere, which may or may not be clinically evident.

282 This term is used to describe the end-stage of renal tuberculosis when all that can be seen is a thin rim of cortical tissue surrounding a large caseous mass in which calcification occurs. The term is inappropriate because it suggests that self-cure has occurred and that the disease has died out whereas in fact live organisms are still liable to be present.

283 Acute tubular necrosis, usually due to 'shock' from any cause, e.g. haemorrhage or acute dehydration. Less common causes of renal failure include renal cortical necrosis, renal papillary necrosis and hypersensitivity to various drugs.

284 The kidneys are enlarged and the cut surfaces bulge due to interstitial oedema and dilatation of the tubules. The cortex is pale because of the absence of blood in the cortical vessels. Microscopically, whereas the glomeruli appear normal, the tubules show varying degrees of destruction, the commonest being tubular epithelial necrosis. The degree and distribution of the tubular damage is variable, more commonly affecting the distal rather than the proximal convoluted tubules.

285 The oliguric or anuric phase in which little or no urine is passed lasts from a few days to four weeks during which both the blood flow through the kidneys and the glomerular filtrate are reduced. Tubular damage results in the non-selective reabsorption of whatever filtrate reaches them. This phase is followed by a diuretic phase during which large volumes of extremely dilute urine are passed. Repair occurs slowly and renal function improves although some permanent impairment may remain.

286 Glomerulonephritis is the term applied to a group of renal diseases where the predominant pathological changes are in the glomeruli and the mechanism is that of either a type III or type II hypersensitivity reaction. They are classified by their light microscopical appearances.

287 Glomerulonephritis is either diffuse, affecting all glomeruli, or focal affecting only some. Focal lesions often show a segmental pattern as well i.e. part of the glomerular tuft being more severely affected than the rest. Diffuse lesions tend to affect the whole glomerulus.

Glomerular reactions by light microscopy are, in broad terms, mixtures of proliferation (increased cellularity) and an increase of extracellular material (i.e. capillary basement membrane and/or mesangial matrix). Hence:
1. diffuse membranous; the cellularity is normal and basement membranes are uniformly thickened
2. diffuse mesangial proliferative; capillaries are normal but there is an increase in mesangial matrix and cells
3. diffuse endocapillary proliferative; there is a great increase in endothelial and mesangial cells which swell the glomerulus and obliterate capillary lumina in some of which polymorphs are seen
4. diffuse mesangiocapillary; increased mesangial cells and matrix with thickening of capillary loops leading to their obliteration
5. focal segmental proliferative; there are increased cells and matrix in parts of the tuft, sometimes with necrosis and usually against a background of diffuse mesangial proliferation
6. diffuse extracapillary; parietal epithelial cells proliferate to form 'crescents'

288 Because they have different natural histories, may have a treatable primary cause (rarely), and respond differently to treatment.

289 Diffuse endocapillary and diffuse mesangial proliferative will usually resolve, the latter not being serious unless it progresses. A quarter of membranous cases will remit spontaneously and the remainder progress through the nephrotic syndrome to chronic renal failure (CRF) slowly, usually over more than 5 or even 10 years. Mesangiocapillary rarely remits and results in CRF more rapidly. Widespread crescent formation is indicative of rapid loss of renal function probably over months and can be seen superimposed on diffuse endocapillary, focal segmental and mesangiocapillary glomerulonephritis.

290 Most cases of glomerulonephritis have no known cause and are therefore idiopathic. Systemic diseases which cause glomerulonephritis are systemic lupus erythematosus, subacute bacterial endocarditis and Henoch-Schönlein purpura. They give rise to a range of changes, the mildest being diffuse mesangial proliferative; the next most severe, focal segmental and the most serious, a superimposed diffuse extracapillary (crescentic) pattern. Polyarteritis nodosa and Wegener's granulomatosis also follow this scheme but are vasculitides, not hypersensitivity, reactions. Membranous and mesangiocapillary glomerulonephritis are predominantly idiopathic though the former may be associated with malignancy, sarcoidosis, hepatitis B surface antigenaemia and penicillamine or gold treatment for rheumatoid disease. Mesangiocapillary glomerulonephritis is sometimes secondary to systemic lupus erythematosus, Henoch-Schönlein purpura or infections such as subacute bacterial endocarditis and infected ventriculo-atrial shunts. Like diffuse endocapillary proliferative, it may also be a post-streptococcal phenomenon. Diffuse mesangioproliferative is rarely idiopathic, and, in addition to the systemic diseases, is seen in IgA nephropathy, a syndrome of recurrent haematuria which is usually self-limiting.

SLE can cause any picture.

291 By immunofluorescence and electron microscopy. They are found where changes are seen on routine light microscopy:
1. in membranous glomerulonephritis in a row outside the glomerular capillary basement membrane
2. in diffuse mesangial glomerulonephritis in the mesangium
3. in mesangiocapillary glomerulonephritis in the mesangium and on the inside of capillary loops

The components in most diseases are usually specific; IgG and C_3 in membranous, C_3 in mesangiocapillary and IgA in IgA nephropathy respectively, but in systemic lupus erythematosus the immunology is mixed whatever the morphology may be.

292 A glomerular disease characterised by no other changes than obliteration of the foot processes of glomerular epithelial cells which can only readily

be seen by electron microscopy. The kidney is thus normal by routine microscopy. Predominantly a disease of children, it gives rise to a selective proteinuria often heavy enough to cause oedema. It responds to steroids and usually stays in remission on their withdrawal.

293 This most commonly takes the form of a diffuse extracapillary proliferation. Immunofluorescence reveals linear deposition of IgG along the capillary basement membrane because this syndrome is a type II hypersensitivity reaction due to antibasement membrane antibodies. Immunofluorescence in all other glomerulonephritides is granular.

294 1. The subcapsular surface of the kidneys is spotted with dark red areas due to congestion and haemorrhage.
2. The renal, segmental and arcuate arteries are atherosclerotic.
3. The intima of the interlobular arteries is thickened by concentric layers of connective tissue (notably elastin) and smooth muscle cells.
4. Fibrinoid necrosis of the wall of the terminal portions of the interlobular arteries and the afferent arterioles occurs and their lumena may be completely blocked. Similar focal necrosis occurs in the glomeruli.
5. A bloody exudate occurs in the capsular space of glomeruli.
6. Some nephrons atrophy and their glomeruli become hyalinised while others enlarge and their tubules dilate and may contain hyaline casts.

295 The kidneys may be normal in size or slightly enlarged. The cortex is pale and the glomeruli may be just visible to the naked eye. Microscopically, diffuse enlargement of the glomeruli is seen and the glomerular capillaries contain only a few red cells which indicates an impaired renal blood flow. This is due to thickening of the capillary walls by an increase in endothelial cell cytoplasm. The underlying cause of these changes is unknown.

296 Other than secondary changes due to hypertension, atherosclerosis and pyelonephritis, which complicate diabetes, the most important specific lesion with a high mortality, particularly in chil-

dren, is diabetic glomerulosclerosis. In this condition there is deposition of eosinophilic hyaline material in the mesangium of the glomerular lobules. The deposits may be nodular or diffuse and if the latter, the appearances are not unlike those of diffuse glomerulonephritis.

297 1. Hyperacute; when the donor kidney has been sensitised to a large number of transplantation antibodies.
2. Acute; such reactions commonly occur within one year of transplantation. The recipient develops a fever, oliguria and tenderness over the affected kidney.
3. Chronic; when the graft ceases to function after a period of months or years. This event is accompanied by hypertension, proteinuria and the appearance of fibrin degradation products in the urine.

298 Lesions develop in both the arteries and renal parenchyma. Gross intimal thickening occurs in the interlobular and arcuate arteries due to the intermittent aggregation of platelets to form thrombi and their incorporation into the wall of the artery. In the renal parenchyma the basement membranes of the glomerular and tubular epithelia become thickened. Immunofluorescent studies demonstrate fine granular deposits of IgM, IgG and complement fractions which outline the capillary walls of the glomeruli and the basement membrane of the tubules.

299 1. Tumours of the renal parenchyma.
    a. Benign. These are common but seldom clinically important. They include adenomata, forming well-defined rounded tumours yellowish in colour, and juxtaglomerular tumours arising from the juxtaglomerular apparatus. They are rare but important since they secrete renin and thus are a rare cause of hypertension.
    b. Malignant. These form 1 per cent of all malignant tumours:
      (i) nephroblastoma, usually occurring before 7 years of age
      (ii) renal adenocarcinoma (hypernephroma)
2. Urothelial tumours arising from the transitional epithelium of the renal pelvis are always malignant.

3. Connective tissue tumours including leiomyomata, fibromata and lipomata are benign and rare.

300 Renal adenocarcinomata arise from the cortex and, if small, tend to project from the upper or lower pole of the affected kidney. The cut surface is usually yellow in colour. Old haemorrhages cause brown patches and necrosis light grey areas. The tumour tends to invade the lumen of the renal vein by direct spread.

Microscopically the tumour cells are arranged in solid trabeculae or in a tubular or papillary fashion. Most of these tumours are composed of characteristic clear cells due to their content of fat and glycogen dissolving out on histological processing.

301 Nephroblastomata account for approximately one-third of all childhood tumours. The maximum age incidence is 3 years and they are seldom encountered after the age of seven. The cut surface of a nephroblastoma is white or greyish white in colour. Cystic spaces may develop as a result of haemorrhage and gelatinous degeneration within the tumour.

Microscopically there is a characteristic mesenchymal stroma composed of spindle cells within which there are primitive, poorly differentiated glomeruli and tubules. Direct spread to adjacent structures is common and blood spread is mainly to lungs, bone and liver.

302 The term hydronephrosis implies that the pelvis and calyces of the kidney have become grossly dilated. If the pelvis is intrarenal, marked atrophy of the renal tissue occurs due to a reduction in the renal blood flow causing ischaemic destruction of the nephrons; first of the tubules and later of the glomeruli. When the pelvis is extrarenal it may dilate considerably with the renal parenchyma remaining intact for a relatively long time. Hydronephrosis occurs as the result of chronic obstruction of the urinary tract at any level from the pelvi-ureteric junction to the external meatus.

303 Pyelonephritis is a bacterial-induced inflammation of the renal pelvis, calyces and renal parenchyma. It is most commonly caused by *E. coli* ascending from the lower urinary tract. It may be acute or

fractures involving the air sinuses may be complicated by infection of the cranium, the subdural or subarachnoid spaces or the brain itself.
3. Aerocoele (pneumatocoele cranii—air under the scalp). An aerocoele develops when bone forming the wall of a paranasal sinus is fractured. If the meninges are torn an aerocoele can rupture into a ventricle.
4. Leakage of cerebrospinal fluid. Cerebrospinal rhinorrhoea may follow a fracture of the frontal, ethmoidal or sphenoidal sinuses whereas a fracture of the temporal bone may be followed by otorrhoea. Infection may supervene in each case.
5. Damage to cranial nerves. Any cranial nerve may be injured if the fracture line involves a foramen. The olfactory nerves are particularly susceptible because of their relatively slender structure.
6. Brain lacerations.
7. Epilepsy. Damage to the cerebral cortex followed by gliosis may result in post-traumatic focal epilepsy.

250 According to the severity of the injury the following may occur:
1. concussion. Unconsciousness immediately following a head injury only occurs if the head moves in response to a blow, thus causing sudden acceleration or deceleration of the brain within the rigid cranium. The opportunity to examine the brain when only transient unconsciousness has occurred is rare but the following pathological changes have been described:
   a. red cells and plasma in the circumvascular (Virchow-Robin) spaces which is a non-specific reaction
   b. axonal 'retraction bulbs', formed from beads of axoplasm which escape after an axon is severed
   c. microglial scars
2. contusion. A contusion is a cluster of more or less confluent petechial haemorrhages associated with variable degrees of necrosis. In a deceleration injury a large contusion may develop at a site diametrically opposite to the point of impact, the so-called 'contrecoup' injury. Small contusions may heal completely

whereas larger ones may be followed by atrophy of the cortex and yellow staining of the pia mater. Microscopic examination reveals gliosis in the affected area and the presence of haemosiderin-containing macrophages, surrounded by a zone of astrocytosis.
3. laceration. This is tearing of cortical surface and overlying pia-arachnoid. Lacerations of the brain are associated with subarachnoid or subdural haemorrhage or gross interstitial haemorrhage.

251 Wallerian degeneration describes the changes which occur when a nerve fibre is separated from its nerve cell.

Within 12 hours fragmentation of the axon can be observed, after which the myelin and the axon form ovoid bodies surrounded by proliferating Schwann cells.

The rate of degeneration is determined by:
1. myelination; heavily myelinated fibres degenerate more rapidly than the unmyelinated
2. function; sensory fibres degenerate faster than motor nerves.

With axonal and myelin degeneration, macrophages, fibroblasts and perineural cells form continuous columns, known as von Bungner's bands. This is the architectural scaffold within which the regenerating axon grows.

At the same time that these changes are taking place distal to the point of section, central chromatolysis occurs in the perikaryon of the parent nerve cell body. This leaves the nerve cell with a thin peripheral rind of Nissl substance. Such changes are not degenerative but merely a response of the nerve cell prior to regenerative activity.

252 1. Lead. Chronic lead poisoning causes dementia probably due to cerebral ischaemia produced by proliferation of the endothelium of the small blood vessels.
2. Mercury. Chronic mercury poisoning causes widespread degeneration in the central nervous system especially in the granular layer of the cerebellar cortex and calcarine area of the cerebral cortex. The classic symptoms of mercury poisoning in the adult are profuse salivation, a coarse tremor and emotional instability. In young children it produces pink disease.

3. Manganese. Chronic manganese poisoning causes loss of neurones in the cerebral cortex, basal ganglia and cerebellum. The result is extra-pyramidal rigidity and a coarse tremor.
4. Tin. This metal is a rare cause of neurological disturbance but the ingestion of organic compounds of this metal causes cerebral oedema.

253 A dysraphic malformation is a congenital abnormality in which the neural tube fails to fuse. Four varieties are recognised:
1. craniorachischis in which the whole neural tube remains open
2. anencephaly when the neural groove of the brain fails to close
3. encephalocoele and meningocoele when failure of closure is limited to the rostral part of the neural tube
4. spina bifida when the defect is limited to the lumbar segments

254 1. Spina bifida occulta. In this condition the vertebral arches of the lumbar region fail to fuse. There is no defect in the spinal cord or roots; the meninges are intact but the site of the defect may be marked in the skin by a dimple, hairy patch or pigmented area.
2. Spina bifida cystica. This may present as:
   a. a meningocoele when a cystic protrusion of the meninges is present beneath the skin but the cord and roots are normal
   b. a myelomeningocoele when the skin over the cyst is absent and the meninges are exposed or even deficient. The arrangement of the cord and nerves is very variable and absence of normal development leads to defective function of the sphincters and paralysis of the lower limbs. A high incidence of hydrocephalus and the Arnold-Chiari malformation are associated with this condition. Infection of the central nervous system eventually occurs if untreated.

255 Down's syndrome is caused by the failure of chromosome 21 to separate during oogenesis with the result that three of these chromosomes are present in a fertilized ovum. Thus the chromosomal composition of a typical Down's baby is 47,XX +21 or 47,XY, +21, this formula indicating the

presence of a male or female with an additional 21 chromosome, a genotype known as trisomy 21. This type of Down's syndrome is commonest in women who bear children towards the end of their reproductive life.

A rarer form of Down's syndrome, not related to maternal age, is associated with 46 chromosomes. One of these is large and is composed of 21 attached to 15, constituting a translocation. Thus the normal complement of chromosomes is present and the trisomy is latent.

256 All are rare. They include:
1. the leucodystrophies
2. the neuronal lipidoses: amaurotic familial idiocy and Niemann-Pick and Gaucher's diseases
3. Phenylketonuria

257 1. Peroneal muscular atrophy (Charcot-Marie-Tooth disease).
2. Friedreich's ataxia.
3. Infantile progressive spinal muscular atrophy (Werdnig-Hoffmann disease).

258 The former is a specific form of degeneration of the central nervous system inherited as a Mendelian dominant and is associated with choreoathetosis and mental deterioration, whereas the latter is a manifestation of acute rheumatic fever in which no specific histological changes in the central nervous system are found.

259 They most commonly develop alongside the superior sagittal sinus following the rupture, due to trauma, of veins in their passage between the arachnoid and dura mater. The bleeding may be so rapid that sudden compression of the underlying brain is produced together with a cerebellar pressure cone followed by death. Alternatively a slow increase in intracranial pressure may occur caused by the liquefaction of a clot and the absorption of fluid into it. The symptoms and signs of the latter are those of an expanding intracranial lesion, usually with marked lateralising signs.

260 The commonest sites for brain haemorrhage are:
1. the lentiform nucleus, due to bleeding from the lenticulostriate branch of the middle cerebral artery

    2. the pons
    3. the white matter of the cerebelllum
The major predisposing factors are:
1. hypertension causing rupture of an atherosclerotic vessel or a microaneurysm
2. A pre-existing brain lesion, e.g. a primary or secondary neoplasm or a septic focus

Death usually occurs following brain haemorrhage due to extension of the haematoma in the cortex or rupture into a ventricle.

261 1. Congenital defects in the media leading to the development of 'berry' aneurysms. Although structural weakness in the media is common the development of an aneurysm is rare. This type of aneurysm most frequently occurs in the middle cerebral artery either at its origin or where it branches.
2. Atherosclerosis.
3. Hypertension.
4. Mycotic, arising in patients suffering from subacute bacterial endocarditis.

262 The middle cerebral, in particular the lenticulostriate branch which supplies that part of the internal capsule which is traversed by the axons of the motor cells in the precentral gyrus as they pass to the cord. Thrombosis of this artery destroys the axons and myelin sheaths in the affected part of the internal capsule resulting in a contralateral hemiplegia. Sensation is preserved because the afferent fibres are situated further back in the internal capsule.

263 Spontaneous thrombosis of the superior longitudinal venous sinus of the brain. It occurs in poorly nourished children who develop an acute infection and in cachetic adults suffering from malignant disease or an infective fever, such as malaria. If the obstruction is complete, intense engorgement of the superficial veins of the brain occurs. This frequently leads to haemorrhagic infarction of the parasagittal areas of the cerebral hemispheres. Thrombosis in the straight sinus causes similar changes in the walls of the third ventricle.

264 The appearance of a cerebral infarct depends upon its age and the associated vascular changes.

    A fresh infarct appears as a swollen area usually ovoid in shape which is softer than the surrounding brain tissue. If necrosis of the vessel walls in the area of the infarct has occurred the infarct is red because of the extravasation of blood from the damaged vessels whereas if the vessels remain intact a pale infarct is produced which, when fresh, may be difficult to distinguish from the normal brain tissue. Within a few weeks the central part of all infarcts liquefies to produce a yellow, gelatinous material which later becomes fluid.

Microscopically, at an early stage, ischaemic necrosis of the neurones occurs. This is followed by the ingress of phagocytes which take up lipid globules derived from myelin degeneration, and haemosiderin from extravasated degenerate erythrocytes. At the periphery, capillary and glial cell proliferation occurs, eventually producing encapsulation.

265 Pachymeningitis is an inflammatory lesion of the dura and leptomeningitis an inflammation of the pia and arachnoid.

Pachymeningitis is rarer than leptomeningitis and is usually caused by the direct spread of infection from the bones of the skull, e.g. following a compound fracture or suppurative otitis media whereas leptomeningitis is caused by organisms carried to the meninges via the blood stream.

266 Gross changes:
1. the dura mater is thickened
2. there may be unilateral or bilateral chronic subdural haematoma
3. the arachnoid mater is thickened and opaque
4. the gyri are atrophied and, in consequence, the sulci are broadened and contain an excess of cerebrospinal fluid
5. the ventricles are enlarged because of cerebral atrophy
6. granular ependymitis occurs

Microscopic changes:
1. the cellularity of the grey matter is increased due to an excess of neuroglial cells
2. the small blood vessels are surrounded by cuffs of lymphocytes and plasma cells
3. the astrocytes are enlarged and branched and are described as 'spider' cells
4. the microglial cells increase in number and may contain iron granules
5. there is neuronal loss

      6. gliosis may be present in the subjacent white matter

267 1. Penetrating injuries of the brain
2. Direct spread of infection from neighbouring septic foci, for example:
   a. temporal lobe abscess following otitis media
   b. cerebellar abscess following mastoiditis
   c. frontal lobe abscess following frontal, ethmoidal or sphenoidal infection
3. Haematogenous infection from:
   a. the lungs, e.g. in bronchiectasis
   b. the heart in infective endocarditis

268 The cytomegalovirus is a herpes virus chiefly affecting newborn babies via the transplacental route. Changes develop in many tissues, the colonised cells becoming greatly enlarged due to distension of the nucleus by inclusion bodies which may also be intracytoplasmic. In infants, death is the result of an encephalitis and children who survive may be mentally retarded or develop hydrocephalus. In adults, many of whom have serological evidence of infection, only a mild or subclinical disease mimicking infectious mononucleosis may occur. This virus is a cause of opportunistic infection in individuals of all ages who are immunodeficient.

269 A disease in which the myelin sheaths of the nerve fibres disappear. This may be a primary phenomenon when, despite the destruction of the myelin sheath, the axon remains at least for a time intact, or it may be secondary in which case the axon is first destroyed with the ensuing disappearance of the myelin.

Primary demyelination follows many viral infections such as measles, varicella, rubella and mumps. A similar condition, post-vaccinial encephalomyelopathy, follows vaccination against smallpox.

Other than infective causes the most important demyelinating disease is multiple sclerosis. The aetiology of this condition remains obscure, laboratory investigation being hindered by the absence of a comparable disease in animals.

270 The commonest pathological change is the development of areas of demyelination, described as plaques. These occur in any part of the central

nervous system but are particularly common in the white matter surrounding the lateral ventricles and in the optic nerves. Plaques of recent origin are yellow or pink in colour and soft in consistency whereas older plaques are grey and firm.

Histology frequently shows the presence of a venule in or near the centre of a recent plaque surrounded by macrophages filled with the lipid breakdown products of myelin. In older lesions the macrophages are surrounded by lymphocytes.

Special stains are required to show the loss of myelin and the proliferation of glial fibres in the plaques.

271 The Lewy body. This is particularly common in the pigmented cells of the substantia nigra and corpora cerulea. These acidophil bodies may be so large that the cell containing them becomes unrecognisable.

272 1. Primary tumours:
  a. neuronal tend to occur in childhood and are malignant; neuroblastoma, medulloblastoma and retinoblastoma
  b. neuroglial are all malignant but variably so
   (i) gliomata are better differentiated histologically and are slower growing. They are named after the cell of origin and include astrocytoma; oligodendroglioma; ependymoma.
   (ii) anaplastic gliomata e.g. glioblastoma multiforme are most malignant
  c. meningioma, commonly benign
  d. nerve sheath and nerve root tumours, all benign
   (i) schwannoma (neurilemmoma, acoustic neuroma)
   (ii) traumatic neuroma
   (iii) neurofibroma may become malignant when multiple (von Recklinghausen's disease)
  e. Uncommon tumours and cysts
   (i) angioma, a developmental malformation
   (ii) haemangioblastoma is malignant
   (iii) epidermoid cyst
   (iv) teratoma, malignant or benign (dermoid cyst)
   (v) craniopharyngioma (supracellar cyst), benign
 2. Secondary tumours are common and may be

chronic and affect one or both kidneys. The condition is commoner in females than males because of the greater incidence of cystitis in the former. In females it is also an important cause of chronic renal failure.

304 1. Sex. It is presumed that pyelonephritis is much commoner in females because infection of the lower urinary tract is commoner in them due to the shorter urethra and trauma to it during sexual intercourse. Nuns have a very low incidence of urinary tract infection compared with sexually active women. Pregnancy may lead to acute bacterial infection of the upper urinary tract due to hormonally induced ureteric atony and dilatation causing urinary stasis.
2. Urinary tract obstruction. This causes infection because:
   a. stagnant urine is a suitable culture media for enteric bacteria
   b. obstruction of the bladder neck predisposes to vesico-ureteric reflux
   c. back-pressure lessens the natural resistance of the kidneys to infection
   d. renal failure caused by chronic obstruction lowers the general resistance of an individual to infection

305 The kidneys are enlarged and oedematous. Radially arranged yellow streaks of pus develop in the medulla and small yellow abscesses eventually occur in the cortex. The pelvic mucosa is thickened, congested and coated with exudate. Microscopically suppurative inflammation is seen in the pelvic submucosa with pus cells in tubules as well as interstitially.

306 Chronic pyelonephritis commonly follows chronic vesico-ureteric reflux and obstructive lesions of the lower urinary tract. The kidneys become shrunken and the surface deformed as the thickness of the renal parenchyma is irregularly reduced. Microscopically, pyogenic abscesses, pus in the tubules and suppuration of the pelvic mucosa may be present. In all cases the glomeruli are sclerosed and replaced by hyalinised collagen. An interstitial chronic inflammatory cell exudate is present but inflammatory changes gradually diminish at the end stage of the disease when the kidney becomes fibrosed.

307 Acute pyelonephritis, diabetes, urinary tract obstruction or the ingestion of analgesic drugs such as aspirin and phenacetin.

308 Congestive, haemorrhagic, bullous, fibrinous, suppurative and gangrenous cystitis describe their macroscopic appearances and their histology corresponds.

309 1. Bacterial infection
2. Metazoal infection, e.g. by *Schistosoma haematobium*.
3. Chemical irritation, e.g. cyclophosphamide.
4. Physical agents such as irradiation.

310 1. Telangiectasia; important because the mucosa may bleed.
2. Progressive fibrosis leading to a reduced bladder capacity.
3. Ulceration of the bladder epithelium leads to severe dysuria.

311 1. Persistent infection within the kidney, e.g. due to a renal calculus, or the presence of a pyonephrosis or tuberculosis of the kidney.
2. Residual urine due to bladder neck obstruction, a diverticulum of the bladder, or malfunction of the bladder caused by a neurological disorder, e.g. multiple sclerosis.
3. The presence of a necrotic tumour.
4. The presence of a bladder calculus.
5. Sexual intercourse is an important cause in females.
6. Certain pH values of the urine, a pH below 5.5 or above 7.5 inhibits the growth of *E. coli*.
7. Osmolality of the urine, a dilute urine inhibits bacterial growth.
8. The presence of glucose in the urine.

312 Hunner's ulceration of the bladder or chronic interstitial cystitis is the name given to a progressive fibrous thickening of the bladder wall accompanied by oedema, lymphatic infiltration and superficial ulceration. Predominantly a disease of females it gives rise to extremely distressing dysuria.

313 Young adult schistosomes pass from the liver down the portal vein to the vesical plexus where mating results in egg production. The eggs cause

granulomatous lesions in the bladder wall. The rectum may be affected similarly.

314 The transitional epithelium lining the infected bladder is ragged and may be ulcerated. The bladder wall is fibrosed and the multinucleate eggs of the metazoan parasite are present in it.

315 1. Chronic inflammation induced either by a retained vesical calculus or *Schistosoma haematobium*.
2. Aromatic amines absorbed through the skin, lungs or alimentary tract which can be metabolised in the liver to 2-amino-1-naphthol, the active carcinogen.
3. Congenital defects; ectopia vesicae.

316 Urothelial tumours of the bladder form either exophytic papillary growths or solid thickening of the wall with a variable degree of ulceration.

317 The microscopic appearance of a vesical tumour depends upon the degree of differentiation. Highly differentiated tumours of low malignant potential consist of papillary projections formed of cells of uniform size and shape which are very regularly arranged. With increasing dedifferentiation, the cells forming the fronds invade the wall and become increasingly irregular in shape and variable in size. Nuclei are hyperchromatic and show numerous mitoses.

GYNAECOLOGY

318 1. Squamous carcinoma is the commonest.
2. Adenocarcinoma was exceedingly rare but a clear-cell variety has been occurring in recent years in teenagers and young women. In many cases, during pregnancy, the mothers of such girls had been treated with synthetic oestrogens which are considered to be the carcinogen.
3. Sarcoma botryoides in young children and the mixed Mullerian tumour which is the adult counterpart. They are both rare and are considered to be a variety of rhabdomyosarcoma.

319 1. Acute: usually non-specific, being caused by staphylococci, streptococci, coliforms etc. This is the result of an abortion, retained products

of conception or, rarely, an intrauterine contraceptive device.
2. Chronic:
   a. non-specific; resulting from the above
   b. specific; usually tuberculous and rarely actinomycotic. Schistosomiasis of the endometrium occurs where that infection is generally endemic.

320 Endometriosis is the presence of normal endometrium (glands plus stroma) in extrauterine sites such as the ovaries, uterine tubes, large bowel, the umbilical skin or abdominal scars and on the serosa of the peritoneal cavity. Adenomyosis, once considered a variety of endometriosis, refers to normal endometrium which is situated deeply in the myometrium.

321 Also known as leiomyofibromata, they are very common benign tumours composed of whorls of smooth muscle and fibrous, collagenous connective tissue. They arise anywhere in the myometrium and when confined to it they are described as mural. If they grow into the uterine cavity or outwards, they are described as submucosal or subserosal, respectively. They occur during the reproductive period and are possibly under some degree of hormonal control.

322 1. Red degeneration which is haemorrhagic infarction.
2. Hyaline degeneration.
3. Calcification. A calcified submucosal fibroid may become detached and passed *per vaginam*—a 'womb stone'.
4. Malignant transformation to leiomyosarcoma is very rare.

323 There are two distinct types:
1. Cystic glandular hyperplasia, or 'Swiss cheese endometrium'. This is due to the action of unopposed oestrogens such as occurs in anovulatory cycles and oestrogen-secreting ovarian tumours. The endometrium is uniformly involved, being thickened, and the glands are well-differentiated. This is not considered to be a particularly pre-malignant condition.
2. Atypical endometrial hyperplasia. This may be combined with the above and usually has the same cause. The changes in the endometrium

are focal and the glandular cells are atypical with hyperchromatic nuclei. Unlike cystic glandular hyperplasia this can be premalignant.

324   1. It is commoner in post-menopausal women, unlike cervical carcinoma.
2. It occurs more often in nulliparous women.
3. In some cases, hyperoestrinism is responsible.
4. There may be focal or diffuse involvement of the endometrium. Both varieties are late in penetrating the myometrium. Spread is directly to the pelvis and later to the extra-pelvic lymph nodes and distant organs.
5. It is an adenocarcinoma which may show evidence of squamous metaplasia. If the last is marked, the growth is described as an adeno-acanthoma. A true adenosquamous carcinoma with a malignant squamous cell element is recognised and has a poor prognosis.
6. With early diagnosis the prognosis is reasonably good, resulting in a 5 year survival rate of 66 per cent.

325   Not an erosion at all but ectopy of the endocervical columnar epithelium which extends beyond the os onto the intravaginal portion of the cervix. Exposure of the epithelium to the acid vaginal contents causes it to undergo squamous metaplasia, thus becoming continuous with the surrounding vaginal epithelium. The cause of the 'erosion' is apparently eversion of the endocervical mucosa due to increase in cervical bulk at puberty, pregnancy, or even possibly during the menstrual cycle.

326   A 'polyp' is a clinical description and not a pathological entity.
1. A mucous polyp is the commonest, consisting of cervical stroma which contains a variable number of cervical glands, some of them distended by mucin.
2. A pedunculated Nabothian follicle; a retention cyst of mucous glands.
3. A squamous papilloma (wart).
4. An exophytic carcinoma.
5. An inflammatory polyp.

327   Nearly all are carcinomata. Nine-tenths are squamous and the remainder adenocarcinomata. Squamous carcinomata are associated with early

and promiscuous sexual activity, early pregnancy and multiple pregnancies. Herpes virus, smegma and DNA from sperm are suspected carcinogens. The disease is uncommon in Jewish women most probably due to circumcision of their male partners rather than to genetic factors. Adenocarcinomata do not appear to be associated with the above causes since they occur more frequently in nulliparous women. They are liable to occur in young girls whose mothers, while bearing them, were treated with oestrogens. Otherwise no other aetiological factors have been identified.

328 The earliest sign of cervical carcinoma is dysplasia of the squamous epithelium as assessed by exfoliative cytology, biopsy or both. In some cases this progresses to *carcinoma-in-situ* and eventually invasive cancer, a process which can take up to fifteen years. Conversely the dysplasia may reverse spontaneously, but since all cases of dysplasia are potentially malignant, the condition is currently described as Cervical Intraepithelial Neoplasia (CIN) and graded 1 to 3, the last being very severe dysplasia, possibly carcinoma-in-situ. The identification of those cases of CIN which are to become malignant is impossible. Dysplasia caused by cervicitis is a complicating factor.

329 1. The stratified squamous epithelial cells show lack of maturation to flat, cornified, glycogen-containing cells.
2. The basal cells form several layers instead of one.
3. There is loss of polarity of the cells which are normally flattened parallel to the surface.
4. The cells become large and variable in size.
5. Nuclei become hyperchromatic and show increased mitotic activity.

330 A large number of tumours occur in the ovary and since the common ones vary in their benign or malignant behaviour, classification does not depend on this.
1. Common epithelial tumours. Nine-tenths are malignant. Many are cystic. Solid or papillary areas in the cyst wall suggest malignancy.
   a. Serous cystadenomata; benign and malignant varieties.
   b. Mucinous cystadenomata; benign and malignant varieties.

c. Brenner tumours; nearly always benign.
 2. Tumours of sex cord-stromal origin.
   a. Granulosa cell tumours; of low grade malignancy and oestrogen secreting.
   b. Theca cell tumours; benign and oestrogen secreting.
   c. Androblastomata, composed of Sertoli or Leydig cells or a mixture of these. Most are benign and most produce virilising (occasionally oestrogenising) hormones.
 3. Germ cell tumours.
   a. Dysgerminoma—very similar in histology, malignancy and radiosensitivity to the seminoma.
   b. Endodermal sinus tumour (yolk sac tumour).
   c. Choriocarcinoma of ovary.
   d. Teratoma; malignant and mature (benign) varieties, the latter described as the dermoid cyst in the past.
 4. Miscellaneous tumours, e.g. fibromata, lipomata, leiomyomata and malignant lymphomata.
 5. Secondary growths, usually from breast, uterus, stomach and large intestine.

331 Ascites and pleural effusions associated with a fibroma of the ovary. This tumour is benign and on its removal, complete cure occurs.

332 Benign:
 a. follicular cysts, including the multiple cysts of the Stein-Leventhal syndrome
 b. corpus luteum cysts, into which haemorrhage may occur
 c. theca-lutein cysts caused by excess gonadotrophins given therapeutically, or due to the presence of a hydatidiform mole
Malignant: these are considered as varieties of ovarian adenocarcinomata.

333 A secondary carcinoma in the ovary which has spread by the transcoelomic route from a gastric or colonic primary.
   Histologically it is composed of signet ring cells in a very cellular stroma which is characteristic and only seen before the menopause. Postmenopausally, the growth looks like a secondary at any site. These tumours are frequently bilateral.

334 1. Hydatidiform mole. The villi are confined to

the endometrium. These tumours are benign but liable to become choriocarcinomata.
2. Invasive mole. This complicates 5 per cent of hydatidiform moles when the villi penetrate the myometrium and even beyond. Emboli of the mole may spread to distant sites. This is benign, the disseminated tissue regressing on excision of the mole. There is no greater chance of choriocarcinoma developing than in a hydatidiform mole.
3. Partial mole. A foetus is usually present but very abnormal and the condition is considered to be due to a chromosomal defect of the conceptus. Most of the placenta is normal but part has the appearance of a hydatidiform mole.
4. Choriocarcinoma. Half of these occur following a mole, quarter after an abortion and a quarter after a normal pregnancy following the retention of products of conception. This is a highly malignant growth and was invariably fatal until the introduction of cytotoxic drugs which now cure 80 per cent of cases.

335 A mass of placental tissue whose villi are exceedingly oedematous thus resembling hydatid cysts. It is the result of trophoblastic proliferation following fertilisation when the ovum later dies. The sperm nucleus with the X chromosome replicates to become diploid and cell division continues to produce the mole. This is borne out by the fact that the mole cells always have two X chromosomes and both are of paternal origin. Although considered benign neoplasms, five per cent become highly malignant choriocarcinomata.

336 The implantation of a fertilised egg and development of the foetus outside the uterus. Nearly all occur in the uterine tubes, mainly the ampulla. Tubal obstruction is usually the reason for this. The pregnancy terminates early, usually after the first missed period, by tubal rupture which causes acute abdominal pain and haemorrhagic shock. Other sites are the ovary or peritoneal cavity.

BREAST

337 1. Amazia: absence of breasts, uni- or bilateral.
2. Athelia: absence of nipples.

    3. Polymastia: additional mammary glands.
    4. Polythelia: additional nipples.

338
1. Fat necrosis, caused by trauma.
2. Inflammation or mastitis:
    a. pyogenic abscess
    b. tuberculosis
    c. plasma cell mastitis (rupture of a cyst or ectatic duct)
    d. fungal and parasitic diseases (rare)
    e. foreign bodies
3. Mammary dysplasia (fibrocystic disease) including single cysts.
4. Primary tumours:
    a. Benign:
        (i) fibroadenoma
        (ii) adenoma (rare)
        (iii) intraduct papilloma
        (iv) phyllodes tumour, also known as cystosarcoma phyllodes or giant fibroadenoma, 20 per cent of which are malignant
        (v) lipoma.
    b. Malignant:
        (i) carcinoma
        (ii) sarcomas, leukaemias and lymphomas are rare
5. Secondary tumours are rare.

339 This is a benign lesion, most commonly occurring in pre-menopausal women. It consists of a variety of alterations of the breast tissue at microscopic level and its cause is unknown. Histology shows any mixture of the following: fibrosis of the stroma, duct ectasia, cyst formation with or without apocrine metaplasia of the cyst lining, adenosis, fibrosing (sclerosing) adenosis, radial scars, epitheliosis, intraduct papillomatosis, ductal hyperplasia and lobular hyperplasia. Some of these conditions are not clear-cut and overlap each other. Subjective interpretation among pathologists is also variable in the case of the proliferative lesions.

340 Recent evidence indicated that those cases with florid proliferation of the epithelial elements (e.g. epitheliosis) have a higher than normal incidence of breast cancer.

341 This is a mixed epithelial and connective tissue

growth and is therefore described as a fibroadenoma. Pure adenomata occur but are rare. Fibroadenomata occur in women younger than those liable to develop carcinoma. They are well-demarcated from the surrounding breast from which they pout when cut across. On microscopy, they consist of well-differentiated glandular structures in a fibrous stroma and have characteristic appearances which cannot be confused with carcinoma. Two varieties, the intracanalicular and pericanalicular are described but many are mixed and there is no clinical significance in this classification.

342 No, but they may recur or be multiple.

343 It is the commonest malignant tumour in women in the affluent countries of the western world.

344 The cause or causes are unknown. Breast cancer is, however, more common in nulliparous than multiparous women. The number of lactations or breast feeding are not important but early maternal age at first pregnancy appears to be protective. There is no evidence for a viral or genetic factor as has been found in mice.

345 There is no generally acceptable classification but the following is currently in use:
1. *in situ* carcinoma
    a. intraduct
    b. intralobular
2. infiltrating carcinoma (corresponding to 1.)
    a. infiltrating duct
    b. infiltrating lobular
       (a mixture of 1. and 2. is often seen).
3. unusual forms:
    a. mucoid (colloid) carcinoma
    b. squamous carcinoma
    c. spindle cell carcinoma
    d. apocrine carcinoma
    e. medullary carcinoma, which is a variety of 2.a. but has a heavy lymphoid cell infiltrate.

346 This is a clinical term used to describe a very fast-growing and rapidly-disseminating cancer of the breast which normally develops during pregnancy or lactation. The skin overlying the tumour is red and oedematous hence the name. It accounts for less than two per cent of all cases of breast cancer.

347 Clinically, it is a chronic eczema of the nipple which may include areola and surrounding skin. Histologically, as well as a non-specific chronic inflammatory cell infiltrate in the dermis, typical Paget cells are seen in the thickness of the dermis. These are large, pale cells with prominent nucleoli occurring singly or in small groups. The epidermis may ulcerate. Underlying the dermal lesion there is a ductal carcinoma of breast, *in situ* or invasive, which may be so small as to require histological examination for detection.

345 Oestrogen receptors are proteins in or on cells to which oestrogens attach themselves thereby inducing the proliferation of these cells. They are therefore present in the cells of organs which are under oestrogen control. This includes normal breast epithelium. Breast carcinoma cells contain variable amounts of receptors and if they are present in appreciable quantities it signifies, firstly, a better prognosis presumably indicating better differentiation and secondly, that the tumours are liable to respond better to anti-oestrogen therapy (drugs and endocrine ablation).

349 Yes. About one per cent of all breast carcinomas arise in males. They have the same histological appearances as in women.

350 They are uncommon. Gynaecomastia, inflammation or carcinoma are the most likely. Gynaecomastia, the commonest swelling in the male breast, may show as diffuse enlargement of the whole breast but is frequently asymmetrical and nodular. One per cent of all mammary carcinomata arise in the male breast.

351 Gynaecomastia, hypertrophy of the male breast, is considered to be due to androgen/oestrogen imbalance. It may thus occur spontaneously at puberty and the climacteric. Otherwise, it is caused by the direct action of oestrogens as is liable to occur in cirrhosis of the liver when normally-present oestrogens are not metabolised. Gynaecomastia may also occur in males with oestrogen-producing tumours, in patients treated by oestrogens for prostatic carcinoma and in men who absorb the hormone while working with it.

The histology is the same whatever the cause. There is an increase in the number of ducts, the epithelial lining of which shows cellular multi-layering, sometimes with papillary projections simulating intraduct carcinoma. The stroma immediately surrounding these ducts has a characteristic oedematous appearance.

MALE REPRODUCTIVE

352 *Escherischia coli*, enterococci, *Proteus mirabilis*, *Pseudomonas aeruginosa* and *Trichomonas vaginalis*. In the past, *Neisseria gonorrhoeae* was the commonest cause.

353 1. Tuberculous.
2. Syphilitic.
3. Fungal.
4. Non-specific.
Non-specific prostatitis is not easily distinguished from carcinoma of the prostate on physical examination. Microscopy reveals tissue infiltrated with a focal or diffuse collection of lymphocytes and plasma cells together with collections of macrophages which resemble the epithelioid cells of tuberculosis. Caseation, however, never occurs.

354 The inner periurethral group of glands.

355 The nodules are composed of hyperplastic glands and fibromuscular stroma. The relative amounts of glandular tissue and stroma varies greatly in different areas and cases. The acini and ducts may contain inspissated secretions, cellular debris and corpora amylaceae. The last are laminated concretions.

356 1. Hypertrophy of the bladder muscle causing trabeculation.
2. The collection of a variable amount of residual urine which eventually becomes infected.
3. Transmission of the increased vesical pressure to the upper urinary tract causes bilateral hydroureter and hydronephroses and, finally, renal failure due to pressure atrophy.
4. Bladder calculi.
5. Diverticula of the bladder. These develop at its base. Once formed, contraction of the bladder tends to increase the distension of the diverticulum which perpetuates its tendency to enlarge.

357 Cancer of the prostate develops in the outer group of prostatic glands, most commonly those situated in the posterior lobe.

358
1. Direct, into the base of the bladder, seminal vesicles and urethra.
2. Lymphatic, to the internal iliac nodes and then upwards, reaching as far as the supraclavicular nodes.
3. Perineural.
4. Haematogenous, mainly to bones, particularly the pelvis, vertebrae, femora or ribs. These lesions may be either osteolytic or osteosclerotic, but usually the latter.

359 Orchitis may be acute, the commonest cause being the mumps virus, or chronic when it may be:
1. tuberculous, either in miliary disease or by direct spread from the epididymis
2. syphilitic, either congenital or acquired. In the latter the commonest lesion is a gumma.
3. granulomatous, in which the testis is wholly replaced by granulation tissue. This condition is now believed to be caused by a reaction in the interstitial tissues of the testes to spermatozoa, the responsible irritant being a lipid.

360
1. Interstitial cell tumours.
2. Sertoli cell tumours.
3. Lymphomata.

361
1. Seminomata are whitish, uniformly soft and well-defined. The tumour is composed of a single type of cell which is large with a rounded, distinct boundary and a clear or faintly granular cytoplasm.
2. Teratomata, the microscopic appearances of which depend upon the histological type. Most have a variegated and cystic appearance with areas of haemorrhage and necrosis. There are four types:
   a. the differentiated or mature teratoma;
   b. the intermediately differentiated or immature teratoma;
   c. the anaplastic teratoma or embryonal carcinoma;
   d. the choriocarcinoma.
3. Combined seminoma and teratoma.

362 A highly malignant tumour occurring in the

gonads of children and young adults. In the testis it is called an orchioblastoma and in the ovary an endodermal sinus tumour. Histologically, it has a typical adenocarcinomatous appearance with cystic spaces and much mucus. It secretes alpha-fetoprotein.

363 Yes; lymphomata account for approximately 10 per cent of testicular tumours. They are most common at 65 years of age, are highly malignant and are frequently associated with lymphomata elsewhere in the body.

364 Teratomata. Raised levels of alpha-fetoprotein (AFP) and Beta human chorionic gonadotrophin (βHCG) are found in the blood of 90 per cent of patients suffering from teratomata.

365 A hard chancre of the penis is caused by the *Treponema pallidum*. It is initially a hard nodule in the coronal region. Superficial or deep ulceration occurs followed by spontaneous healing within 30–60 days. In all cases marked inguinal lymphadenopathy occurs. Microscopically there is an initial collection of polymorphonuclear leucocytes which is soon replaced by lymphocytes and plasma cells, tending to be most prominent around the blood vessels.

366 Erythroplasia of Queyrat and Bowen's disease which are essentially examples of carcinoma *in situ*. In both, acanthosis and hyperkeratosis occur together with varying degrees of dysplasia, constituting the *in situ* phase which progresses to invasive malignancy.

367 Fournier's gangrene is an infection of the skin and subcutaneous tissue covering the testes. It is caused by a mixed infection with haemolytic streptococci and bacterioides. It spreads with remarkable rapidity and if untreated it leaves the testicles devoid of skin.

368 Carcinoma of the skin of the scrotum in chimney sweeps, described by Sir Percival Pott in 1775. The same tumour (known as mule spinner's cancer) was also observed to occur in the groin region in men exposed to the shale oil which is sprayed from the spinning mule.

ENDOCRINE SYSTEM

369 A craniopharyngioma is a rare tumour derived from misplaced cells of the hypophyseal recess, Rathke's pouch, during development. The tumour is both solid and cystic. The solid areas consist of islets of squamous epithelium in a loose stroma of stellate cells and the tumour thus resembles an adamantinoma. The cystic spaces are lined by keratinised squamous epithelium and are filled with clear or turbid straw-coloured fluid which contains cholesterol crystals.

370 Sheehan's syndrome consists of infarction of the pituitary gland following parturition which is complicated by severe haemorrhage. Survival of the acute episode is followed by chronic pituitary insufficiency (Simmond's disease) the chief features of which are weakness, loss of energy, anhidrosis, myxoedema, loss of libido and amenorrhoea. Each is due to lack of the respective hormones produced by the pituitary.

371 Ten per cent of all intracranial tumours arise from the adenohypophysis. In order of frequency, 70 per cent arise from the chromophobe cells, 25 per cent from the acidophil cells and five per cent from the basophil cells.

372 The clinical effects of tumours of the adenohypophysis are usually caused by pressure atrophy of the gland by a chromophobe adenoma which produces hypopituitarism. Some of these adenomata secrete trophic hormones, the commonest being prolactin. An acidophil adenoma causes acromegaly and gigantism due to growth hormone secretion and a basophil adenoma, Cushing's disease.

373 Diabetes insipidus is caused by the lack, or failure of release of, the hormone vasopressin from the posterior lobe of the pituitary. No obvious lesion is usually present, but a primary tumour of the hypothalamus or the presence of metastases in this region must be excluded.

374 Acromegaly is due to an increased secretion of growth hormone after normal bone growth has ceased and is caused by an acidophil adenoma of the adenohypophysis. The features of the face

become coarser because of thickening of the skin and subcutaneous tissue. The skull may enlarge and the lower jaw protrude. The paranasal sinuses increase in size causing prominence of the supraorbital ridges and the tongue enlarges as does the larynx. There is enlargement of the hands and feet and osteoarthrosis of the weight-bearing joints occurs. Diabetes is common because the excess growth hormone antagonises the action of insulin. If bone growth has not ceased, gigantism occurs.

375 1. Diffuse are more commonly benign than malignant. The patient may be euthyroid, toxic or myxoedematous.
2. Multinodular goitres may be benign or malignant and over-active or normal in function.
3. Solitary nodules may be benign or malignant and are occasionally active.

376 A multinodular goitre consists of numerous nodules, which are the result of foci of hyperplasia, separated by bands of collagen. Some of these foci undergo colloid change whereas in others haemorrhage occurs leading to necrosis and cyst formation. Both fibrosis and calcification can occur in the degenerate nodules.

377 A simple goitre consists of a generalised enlargement of the thyroid gland without evidence of under- or over-activity. Histologically a simple goitre is composed of enlarged vesicles filled with colloid and lined by a flattened epithelium.

378 1. A dietary deficiency of iodine.
2. An increased demand for thyroid hormones, e.g. in pregnancy, producing a physiological goitre.
3. A congenital enzyme defect which either interferes with the uptake of iodine by the gland or the synthesis of thyroxine. This is a dyshormogenic goitre.
4. Chemical agents which interfere with thyroxine synthesis, e.g. para-aminosalicylic acid, thiouracil, carbimazole and substances occurring in vegetables of the brassica family (cabbage and turnips).

379 Primary thyrotoxicosis is an organ-specific autoimmune disease most probably caused by the presence in the serum of an immunoglobulin,

human thyroid stimulating antibody. This is believed to displace TSH from binding sites on the thyroid follicle membrane thus causing prolonged stimulation of thyroid activity. The physiological effects of thyroid stimulation are the excessive secretion of two thyroid hormones, T_3 and T_4. The former is only a small fraction of the circulating thyroid hormone but it has a substantial calorigenic effect because it is less well bound to the plasma proteins which carry it.

380 In an untreated toxic goitre the thyroid follicles are lined by a hyperplastic epithelium which produces papillary infoldings into the follicles. The cells are larger than normal and the amount of colloid is reduced. Clear spaces are seen in the watery pale-staining colloid at the margin of the follicle giving it a characteristic scalloped appearance.

Following treatment with iodine the colloid stores are replenished but if anti-thyroid drugs, such as carbimazole, are administered, the hyperplasia and infolding of the epithelium increases. Commonly there is some degree of lymphoid infiltration of the thyroid, usually diffusely scattered throughout the gland but sometimes focal.

381 A toxic adenoma is a true adenoma of the thyroid which has become so active that the patient suffers from thyrotoxicosis. Ocular symptoms are absent and immunoglobulins are not present in the serum. Due to normal feed-back mechanisms a 'hot' nodule suppresses TSH production with the result that the remaining glandular tissue becomes inactive.

382 1. Hashimoto's disease (lymphadenoid goitre).
2. Primary myxoedema.
3. Focal thyroiditis.
In all of these, antibodies to thyroglobulin and the microsomes of the follicular epithelial cells occur in the serum. Other auto-immune diseases such as atrophic gastritis and Addison's disease may be present.

383 The thyroid in Hashimoto's disease is enlarged symmetrically or asymmetrically. The surface is smooth. The gland is greyish white in colour and the cut surface is uniform. One striking feature is the avascularity of the gland.

Microscopically the most distinctive features is the intense lymphocytic and plasma cell infiltration. Foci of these may contain lymphoid follicles. In the late stages, remaining thyroid follicles are small and contain only minimal quantities of colloid. The follicular epithelial cells become large and irregular with eosinophilic cytoplasm and are known as Askanazy cells.

384 The precise cause of Riedel's thyroiditis is unknown. Some pathologists regard it as the fibrotic end stage of Hashimoto's disease. However, whereas myxoedema commonly occurs in Hashimoto's, it is never seen in Riedel's disease. The gland is extremely hard and the margins ill-defined because the fibrous tissue replacing the normal tissue infiltrates the overlying strap muscles. Microscopy shows that the parenchyma of the gland is replaced by dense collagen which contains a few scattered, shrunken follicles together with a cellular infiltrate consisting of lymphocytes, plasma cells, neutrophils and eosinophils.

385 Tumours of the thyroid may be:
1. Benign:
   a. microfollicular adenoma
   b. foetal adenoma
   c. Hürthle cell adenoma
2. Malignant: these are rare, accounting for 0.3 per cent of all cancer deaths:
   a. papillary carcinoma
   b. follicular carcinoma
   c. anaplastic carcinoma
   d. medullary carcinoma
   e. squamous cell carcinoma
   f. miscellaneous tumours including malignant lymphoma and teratoma

386 1. The tissue is commonly solitary and well-encapsulated.
2. Microscopically the tumour consists of numerous follicles and a varying number of solid masses of cells. Oxyphilic (Hürthle) cells forming solid sheets make up a large part of the tumour.
3. The diagnosis of malignancy is confirmed by finding capsular and/or vascular invasion.

387 1. It is rarely encapsulated.
2. Multiple foci of tumour are visible to the naked

eye in 20 per cent and microscopically in 85 per cent.
3. The tumour may contain psammoma bodies.
4. Microscopically papillary projections are seen in the colloid-filled follicles.
5. The tumour rarely spreads via the bloodstream but may be found in adjacent lymph nodes.

388
1. In 20 per cent of patients this tumour is familial forming one part of the multiple endocrine neoplasia II complex.
2. The tumour arises from the calcitonin-secreting parafollicular C-cells.
3. Whereas the sporadic tumour is unilateral, in familial cases it is frequently bilateral and multifocal.
4. The tumour or tumours are discrete and greyish in colour.
5. Microscopically the tumour consists of small undifferentiated cells with amyloid in the stroma.
6. The tumour metastasises to the regional lymph nodes and later to the skeleton, liver and lungs.

389
1. Chronic renal failure, the common causes of which are chronic glomerulonephritis, chronic pyelonephritis, polycystic disease of the kidneys and hydronephrosis.
2. Malabsorption.

390
1. Primary due to:
   a. the presence of single or multiple adenomata
   b. hyperplasia of the water clear cells or chief cells
   c. carcinoma of the parathyroid
2. Secondary due to compensatory hyperplasia of the parathyroid glands in response to a fall in the ionised serum calcium, low serum magnesium or low vitamin D concentration.
3. Tertiary caused by the development of adenomata in the hyperplastic glands of secondary hyperparathyroidism, most frequently seen in chronic renal failure due to failure of vitamin D synthesis. This is no longer compensatory as in 2. and is manifest by a rising serum calcium.

391
1. The formation of calculi, consisting chiefly of calcium phosphate, in the urinary tract.
2. Nephrocalcinosis.

3. Metastatic calcification in various tissues, in particular, the walls of arterioles.
4. Demineralisation of the skeleton. Loss of calcium from bone leads to a decrease in bone density which can be seen radiologically.
5. Osteitis fibrosa cystica, von Recklinghausen's disease of bone.
6. Peptic ulceration.
7. Acute pancreatitis.
8. Arthropathy due to the deposition of calcium in joint cartilage.

392 The islet cells of the pancreas belong to the APUD system. There are three types in the human pancreatic islets:
1. alpha cells which secrete glucagon
2. beta cells secreting insulin
3. delta cells which secrete gastrin
In general, tumours of the cells of the APUD system, apudomata, may secrete 'inappropriate' hormones, i.e. hormones not produced by the normal cells. Thus an insulinoma may secrete in addition to insulin, secretin, ACTH, melanocyte stimulating or antidiuretic hormone.

393 The Zollinger-Ellison syndrome is caused by the excessive secretion of gastrin by delta cell tumours of the pancreatic islets, 60 per cent of which are malignant, or by hyperplasia of the gastrin-secreting cells of the pylorus of the stomach. This causes hypersecretion of hydrochloric acid resulting in intractable multiple peptic ulcers in the duodenum and upper jejunum. The alkaline secretion of the pancreas is neutralised causing severe diarrhoea and the inactivation of the pancreatic enzymes leads to steatorrhoea.

394 Bacterial or viral infections, pregnancy, severe trauma and disseminated intravascular coagulation. Acute destruction is followed by severe hypotension, cyanosis and death. The classic syndrome, the Waterhouse-Friderichsen, occurs following infection with *Neisseria meningitides*.

395 In the past chronic destruction of the adrenal glands was due to tuberculosis or mycotic infections. In the UK today the most common causes of adrenal destruction are replacement by secondary malignant tumours, auto-immunity or amyloidosis usually associated with rheumatoid

arthritis. Chronic destruction leads to Addison's disease.

396 Addison's disease is due to chronic destruction of the adrenal cortex from whatever cause. It is characterised by increasing fatigue, muscular weakness, abdominal discomfort and brown pigmentation of the buccal mucosa and the areas of skin exposed to light. This last change is due to the melanocyte stimulating action of corticotrophin which is produced in increased amounts by the pituitary. The deficiency of cortisol causes an imbalance of sodium ions and water between the intra- and extracellular compartments and thus hypotension.

397 Non-chromaffin tumours of the adrenal medulla are of two types:
1. neuroblastoma (sympathicoblastoma). This is malignant and occurs in infancy and childhood. It forms a large purple-grey tumour in which haemorrhagic and necrotic areas occur. Microscopically, clusters, sheets or rosettes of small round or oval cells are present. The centres of the rosettes are occupied by pink-staining neurofibrils.
2. ganglioneuroma. This is benign, occurs in young adults and forms firm lobulated encapsulated masses, the cut surfaces of which may have a whorled appearance. The tumour is composed of Schwann cells, reticulin fibres, collagen and irregular bundles of nerve fibres together with groups of mature ganglion cells.

398 A phaeochromocytoma is a chromaffin tumour of the adrenal medulla or extra-adrenal chromaffin tissues. Such tumours are occasionally part of the multiple endocrine syndrome. They form greyish-brown masses in which cystic and haemorrhagic areas may be seen. Microscopically the tumour is similar to normal adrenal medulla consisting of groups of irregularly-shaped cells enclosed in a fine framework of reticulin and collagen fibres.

These tumours secrete excessive amounts of adrenaline and noradrenaline which cause a variety of symptoms including those resulting from the severe hypertension which the hormone produces.

399 1. Virilism causing sexual precocity in boys and pseudohermaphroditism in girls.

2. Feminisation leading to sexual precocity in girls and feminisation of the male.
3. Aldosteronism.
4. Cushing's syndrome; obesity, a 'moon face', the buffalo hump, protein loss and thinning of the abdominal skin leading to the development of purple striae, osteoporosis and diabetes in many patients.

400 Cushing's syndrome is due directly to the excessive secretion of corticosteroids by an adrenal cortical adenoma, a carcinoma or adrenal hyperplasia whereas Cushing's disease is caused by excess secretion of ACTH by a pituitary basophil adenoma resulting in the secretion of cortisone by the stimulated adrenal.

401 Conn's syndrome is due to the excessive secretion of aldosterone by the adrenal cortex, the result of cortical hyperplasia, a cortical adenoma or, rarely, a carcinoma. This causes a number of biochemical abnormalities including a low plasma renin, intermittently lowered serum calcium, hypokalaemia, hypernatraemia and impaired glucose tolerance. The clinical manifestations are polyuria, polydipsia and periodic muscular weakness.

402 These syndromes are characterised by hyperplastic or neoplastic proliferation of more than one endocrine gland. There are three types, all apparently inherited as autosomal dominants. MEN I (Werner's syndrome) consists of adenomata of the pituitary, pancreatic islets and parathyroid glands although the last usually shows only chief cell hyperplasia. Adenomata of the adrenal cortex and thyroid may also be present. MEN II (Sipple's syndrome) is typified by medullary carcinoma of the thyroid, phaeochromocytoma and parathyroid chief cell hyperplasia.

MEN III (MEN IIB or Gorlin's syndrome) consists of medullary carcinoma of the thyroid, phaeochromocytoma, mucosal neuromata (especially of the lips), skeletal abnormalities and a marfanoid habitus.

SKIN

403 Although both are non-specific pyogenic infections of skin, the former, better known as a boil,

is a localised abscess which has started in a hair follicle. The latter is a spreading infection of the dermis with indistinct, irregular margins, which may discharge pus at several points on the skin surface.

404 Impetigo is a suppurative inflammation of the superficial skin where intra-epidermal bullae and pustules form. The causative organisms are staphylococci. Erysipelas is a cellulitis of the dermis cause by *Streptococcus pyogenes*. The latter may, very occasionally, lead to the post-streptococcal conditions, acute rheumatic fever and acute glomerulonephritis.

405 Dermatitis is a clinical term used to describe an inflammatory lesion of the skin caused by a large variety of agents e.g. contact with an irritant or a hypersensitivity reaction to an exogenous or endogenous antigen. It is synonymous with eczema.

406 In acute dermatitis the keratinocytes are separated by intercellular oedema within which lymphocytic infiltration occurs. Degeneration and liquefaction of the cells leads to the formation of vesicles within the epidermis which then rupture onto the surface producing a 'weeping' area. In the dermis varying degrees of oedema, vascular dilatation and congestion occur together with a perivascular cellular infiltrate consisting of lymphocytes, eosinophils and leucocytes. In contrast, in chronic dermatitis the epidermis shows marked acanthosis with elongation of the rete ridges. No vesicles are present and only a moderate cellular infiltrate occurs. The result is a skin of leathery appearance.

407 Although these virus groups are structurally different, both produce a blister which histologically appears as an intra-epidermal vesicle. The epidermal cells attacked by the viruses undergo a series of changes:
1. enlargement
2. the development of an eosinophilic cytoplasm
3. vacuolation
4. loss of adhesion or acantholysis, so that the cells lie loose in the bullae
5. the presence within the cells of inclusion bodies which, in smallpox, are cytoplasmic and

in herpes simplex, zoster and chickenpox, intranuclear

408 Yes. Circulating antibodies to some constituent of the intercellular region of keratinocytes may be demonstrable in the serum in active disease. Such antibodies bound to complement may be demonstrated by direct or indirect immunofluorescence. In dermatitis herpetiformis deposits of IgA may be found in the dermal papillae.

In bullous pemphigoid, linear deposits of IgG may be found bound to the basement membrane of the stratified squamous epithelium.

409 'Fish-skin disease' is the lay term for an inherited disease of the skin known dermatologically as ichthyosis, in which the skin is dry and scaly due to marked hyperkeratosis. Two types occur, one an autosomal dominant type which occurs in both sexes and a second, a sex-linked recessive type occurring only in males. In the former, marked thinning of the granular layer occurs and in the latter, marked hypertrophy.

410 1. Parakeratosis, the extent and degree depending upon the chronicity of the lesion.
2. Absence of the granular layer.
3. Acanthosis of the epidermis with elongation of the rete ridges and narrowing of the suprapapillary epidermis.
4. Slight inflammatory infiltration of the dermis.

411 A sebaceous cyst (pilosebaceous cyst or wen) is formed in a hair follicle, possibly due to obstruction at the skin surface. The hair substance continues to be secreted together with sebum from the associated sebaceous gland, the last eventually suffering pressure atrophy. The cyst is lined by stratified squamous epithelium and the contents are greasy keratin.

An epidermoid cyst is considered to be the result of sequestration of epidermis at a fusion line during foetal development.

A dermoid cyst or dermoid inclusion results from traumatic inoculation of epidermis into the dermis where the epithelium forms a cyst and continues to secrete keratin.

The gross and histological appearances of all three are similar although fine differences such as absence of an associated sebaceous gland are described in the last two.

412 Acne vulgaris commences at puberty and affects males and females equally. The initial abnormality is a blockage of the openings of the pilosebaceous follicles by keratinous debris, and affects chiefly the follicles of the face, chest and upper back although in severe cases it may become more extensive. The deposition of bacteria, debris and possibly melanin in the superficial part of the keratin plug forms the typical 'blackhead' and the keratinous plug as a whole is known as the comedo.

In the second stage the contents of the follicle become infiltrated with polymorphonuclear leucocytes and eventually pus is discharged onto the surface. Secondary infection can occur with *Corynebacterium acnes*, a commensal anaerobic diphtheroid organism which can split the neutral fat in the sebum into free fatty acids. These are extremely irritating to the surrounding tissues and if the follicular wall disintegrates a perifolliculitis develops which, on healing with fibrosis, causes disfigurement. The precise cause of acne remains to be elucidated but the hormonal changes associated with puberty are believed to be at least partially responsible.

413 Tumours of the epidermis can be benign or malignant.
   1. Benign:
      a. squamous and basal cell papillomata. The latter tend to occur in the elderly and form pigmented, greasy, warty growths. They are also known as senile seborrhoeic warts.
      b. naevi or moles, which arise from the melanocytes normally present in the basal cells of the epidermis
      c. a group of tumours, usually benign, which arise from epidermal appendages, usually sweat glands, e.g. syringoma and hidradenoma
   2. Malignant:
      a. squamous carcinoma
      b. basal cell carcinoma
      c. intra-epidermal squamous carcinoma otherwise known as *carcinoma-in-situ* or Bowen's disease
      d. malignant melanoma
      e. secondary tumours, having spread from tumours elsewhere in the body. They usually develop in the dermis and eventu-

ally ulcerate the epidermis. In the case of Paget's disease of the nipple, the tumour cells are found in the epidermis

414 A wart is a viral-induced benign neoplasm caused by one of approximately 30 strains of DNA papovirus. It consists of an irregular overgrowth of the stratum spinosum of the epidermis, described as acanthosis. Basophilic granules in these cells are considered to be the viral particles. A viral cause of the wart is also indicated by vacuolation round the nuclei of the wart cells which are then described as koilocytes.

415 Both are warty growths on the skin in perineal and genital areas and have an infective aetiology. Condylomata lata constitute one of the lesions of secondary syphilis. They contain *Treponema pallidum*, are highly infective and are not considered to be neoplasms. Condylomata acuminata are, however, classified with the warts of the skin and are considered to be neoplasms. They are caused by a DNA virus but like the lata, they are venereal infections and are known as venereal warts. They are large and cauliflower-like whereas the lata are smaller and form flat papules. Venereal warts may, rarely, become malignant, indicating their neoplastic nature.

416 A keratoacanthoma, also known as molluscum sebaceum, is a tumour-like but self-healing lesion which predominantly occurs on the face of adults. Typically the lesion forms a nodule which rapidly enlarges over several weeks to form a mass one to two centimetres in diameter. As growth occurs the lesion becomes umbilicated and when growth ceases the central depression enlarges and the central plug is discharged, the whole process taking several months.

Histologically, the cells of the lesion resemble squamous carcinoma cells and are often indistinguishable from them. A section of the whole lesion, however, indicates its nature by its characteristic flask-shape as it bulges out from the surrounding skin and lifts up the adjacent normal skin margins. Fragmentation of the lesion at excision must be avoided for satisfactory histological examination.

417 It consists of an eruption of waxy, skin-coloured

papules with a characteristic central umbilication and is caused by infection with a DNA pox virus. The lesions consist of a localised proliferation of the epidermis into the dermis compressing the connective tissue which forms a pseudo-capsule. The basal cells contain small oval eosinophilic inclusion bodies which become basophilic as the cells degenerate. The molluscum bodies are composed of aggregations of virus particles which are infective.

418 1. The benign variety includes non-related lesions such as the xanthoma which is a pseudo-tumour. Most of them, however, are considered to be related to each other and constitute a spectrum. They usually occur in the dermis and are described either as dermatofibromata or histiocytomata. Sclerosing haemangioma is an outmoded name for the former when it contains many small blood vessels, some thrombosed, and haemosiderin. These tumours are slow-growing.
2. Fibrous histiocytoma of intermediate malignancy—the dermatofibrosarcoma protuberans.
3. Malignant fibrous histiocytoma.

The essential cellular features of all of the above are:
1. a histiocytic origin indicated by electron microscopy and immunohistochemistry
2. multinucleate cells
3. a 'storiform' or cartwheel arrangement of the cells

419 A rodent ulcer, so-called because it erodes tissues, is also known as a basal cell carcinoma. It can arise on any part of the skin except the palms and the soles but most usually occurs on the face. Sunlight predisposes to its development. Histologically, the growth consists of islets of cells whose appearances are similar to those of the basal cells of the epidermis. Characteristic palisading occurs round the islets. The tumour grows locally, causing ulceration of the skin and invading the dermis and subcutaneous structures. Metastasis does not occur and local excision or x-irradiation are successful treatments.

420 Squamous carcinoma can arise anywhere on the skin but parts exposed to sunlight are most vulnerable. It begins as a scaly or warty lesion and

then ulcerates. Typically the ulcer has a rolled edge. Extension to surrounding skin and deep tissues occurs and lymphatic spread to local lymph nodes causes them to enlarge. Lymphatic and blood spread to distant organs then occurs.

Histologically, in the early stages the malignant transformation may occur while the cells are still in the epidermis (*carcinoma-in-situ* or Bowen's disease). The cells become variable in size and lose their polarity. Mitotic activity increases and there is increased keratin production on the surface. Individual epidermal cells show dyskeratosis i.e. keratinisation. With invasion, irregular islets of the cancer cells infiltrate and destroy normal tissue. The tumour may be well-differentiated when epithelial pearls consisting of prickle cells surrounding mature keratin flakes are seen, or poorly-differentiated consisting of oval cells which are difficult to recognise as being of squamous epithelial origin.

421   1. Mongolian spot or blue naevus when melanocytes remain in the dermis instead of migrating to epidermis.
2. An ephelis (freckle) where the normal numbers of melanocytes present among the basal cells of the epithelium produce increased amounts of melanin.
3. Lentigo where a focus of continuous melanocytes are present beneath the basal layer of the epithelium.
4. Naevus or naevus-cell mole.
   a. junctional
   b. intradermal
   c. compound
   The overlying skin may be warty and the lesion is considered to be a hamartoma rather than a neoplasm.
5. Malignant melanoma
   a. lentigo maligna
   b. superficial spreading melanoma
   c. nodular melanoma
   a. and b. may be considered *melanoma in situ* since they grow horizontally but sooner or later they invade deeply to form a nodular melanoma.

422   There are three types of malignant melanoma, the first two described below being malignant melanoma-in-situ since they do not invade or metas-

tasize although they have this potentiality. If and when they invade into the dermis they become nodular melanomata.

1. Lentigo maligna or Hutchinson's freckle is flat and arises on areas of the skin exposed to the sun. The basal layer of the epidermis is replaced by rather bizarre melanocytes which may proliferate or regress and the freckle thus moves about the skin to some extent. This may persist for 20 years before becoming invasive, forming a nodular melanoma which has a good prognosis.

Acral lentiginous and mucosal melanomata have been described separately. They occur on the palms, soles and mucosae and although they resemble lentigo maligna histologically, they have a worse prognosis than superficial spreading melanoma.

2. Superficial spreading melanoma is slightly raised, can occur anywhere on the skin and becomes a nodular melanoma in about 7 years. As in 1, melanocytes replace the basal layer of epithelium but are much more dysplastic and bizarre and they infiltrate the full thickness of the epidermis towards the surface. The prognosis is between that of 1 and 2.

3. Nodular melanoma is invasive *ab initio*, the malignant melanocytes spreading both into the dermis and deeper tissues and upwards into the epidermis. Even when adequately excised locally, prognosis is related to depth of invasion, ulceration of the skin, mitotic rate and, of course, lymphatic permeation.

BONES & JOINTS

423 1. *Staphylococcus aureus*, causing acute, subacute and chronic osteomyelitis.
2. *Mycobacterium tuberculosis*, causing chronic osteomyelitis.
3. *Mycobacterium lepri*, commonly affecting the terminal phalanges directly or, by causing a peripheral neuropathy, producing neuropathic joints.

424 Bone may be infected directly following a compound fracture, or indirectly via the blood stream from an infective focus elsewhere in the body, e.g. a boil or furuncle. Acute osteomyelitis

due to haematogenous spread occurs in children and is frequently preceded by injury to the affected bone, most commonly the metaphyseal ends of the femur or tibia. The organism, carried in an infected embolus, reaches a metaphyseal end-artery and the bone supplied by the artery becomes infected and necrotic. A rapidly developing inflammatory response causes increased intraosseous tension which causes not only severe pain but also compression of adjacent blood vessels which increases necrosis.

Finally, as pus reaches the surface of the cortical bone it strips the periosteum from it. This interrupts the periosteal blood supply to the bone with the result that the whole thickness of the cortex dies. Simultaneously the periosteum begins to form new bone, known as the involucrum, which is usually perforated by a large cloaca and through which pus reaches the surface.

Since dead bone is only slowly resorbed, in the pre-antibiotic era acute osteomyelitis often became chronic and numerous sinuses developed in the skin through which pus and necrotic pieces of bone were discharged.

425 *Streptococcus haemolyticus, Streptococcus pneumoniae, Haemophilus influenzae, Escherichia coli* and organisms of the salmonella group.

426 Pott's disease is caused by infection of the vertebrae by *Mycobacterium tuberculosis*. Destruction of the intervertebral discs and adjacent bodies of the vertebrae causes them to collapse, producing the characteristic angular kyphos. Caseous material from the vertebral lesion may compress the cord to cause paraplegia, and, gaining access to the psoas sheath, it may spread downwards to present subcutaneously below the inguinal ligament at the inner aspect of the thigh as a psoas abscess.

427 Failure to produce mature collagen leading to:
1. spongy, bleeding gums and loss of teeth
2. the breakdown of old wounds

428 1. An inadequate intake; to prevent rickets a daily intake of 400 i.u. is required, to prevent osteomalacia 100 i.u.
2. Inadequate absorption.
3. Inadequate synthesis in the body due to lack of exposure to ultraviolet light.

429 Rickets is a metabolic disorder of bone caused by a deficiency of Vitamin D in infancy or childhood. The organic matrix of the bone, i.e. osteoid, is not mineralised. The bones are, therefore, soft and liable to become deformed.

430 The long bones of the lower limbs, pelvis, ribs and skull. Softening of the weight-bearing long bones leads to bowing of the legs. Softening of the pelvis leads to transverse compression. Involvement of the epiphyseal cartilages of the ribs causes enlargement of the costochondral junctions producing the 'rachitic rosary'. In the skull, bossing of the frontal and parietal bones occurs and the anterior fontanelle is late in closing.

431 1. Failure of mineralisation of the osteoid matrix and the cartilage of epiphyseal plates.
2. Persistence of hyperplastic cartilage cells in the epiphyseal plates causing the plates to become thicker and wider.
3. Failure of metaphyseal modelling because uncalcified osteoid is not easily reabsorbed by osteoclasts.

The combination of 2. and 3. results in the flared metaphyses and irregular growth plates characteristic of rickets.

432 Failure of osteoid calcification, osteoid being increased at the expense of mineralised bone. This can be demonstrated by staining a trephine biopsy of the iliac crest by von Kossa's or Goldner's method. The former stains mineral (calcium salts) black/brown and leaves the osteoid unstained, the latter stains mineralised bone blue and osteoid orange. In osteomalacia, wide bands of osteoid are shown at the margin of bony trabeculae.

433 1. A normal or lowered serum calcium.
2. A low serum phosphate.
3. Elevated alkaline phosphatase.
4. Aminoaciduria.

434 1. Bone pain.
2. Skeletal deformity—producing kyphosis, distortion of ribs and bending of the pubic rami.
3. Muscular weakness.

435 Osteosclerosis is a condition in which an increase

in bone mineralisation causes the trabeculae to be thickened, but despite this the affected bones are more fragile than normal. A common cause is metastatic carcinoma from the prostate. Less common causes include:
1. chronic renal failure
2. fluorosis from the continuous intake of highly fluoridinated water
3. a rare metabolic disease of bone known as Albers-Schönberg disease (osteopetrosis or marble bone disease)

436 Osteoporosis is a condition in which the bone mass decreases due to the rate of bone resorption exceeding that of formation.

437 1. Endocrine disturbances, the commonest of which is the postmenopausal deficiency of oestrogens and, less commonly, Cushing's syndrome, corticosteroid over-administration and thyrotoxicosis.
2. Reflex osteoporosis such as Sudeck's astrophy of the bones of the hand, wrist and forearm following a Colles' fracture.
3. Inflammation; any type of inflammatory lesion in bone is accompanied by localised peri-inflammatory osteoporosis, e.g. around fracture sites.
4. Disease which causes prolonged immobilisation, e.g. following motor paralysis.
5. Liver disease; cirrhosis may eventually cause osteoporosis.
6. Lack of gravity as occurs in space flight.

438 1. Thinning of the cortical bone.
2. Narrowing of the trabeculae and a reduction in their number.
This decrease in the total mass of mineralised tissue is unaccompanied by qualitative changes.

439 An increased incidence of fractures particularly in females who have a smaller bone mass than males. The commonest fractures are of the neck of the femur and the lower ends of the radius and ulna. Weakness of vertebrae results in progressive kyphosis.

440 This is a collective term describing the skeletal complications of chronic renal failure.
These include: osteomalacia, osteitis fibrosa due

to secondary hyperparathyroidism, osteoporosis and osteosclerosis.

441 Osteochondrosis is a condition in which one or more epiphyses become necrotic and fragmented due to defective blood supply. It may be associated with:
1. injury to an epiphysis
2. endocrine disturbance e.g. Fröhlich's syndrome
3. renal osteodystrophy
4. Gaucher's disease

A number eponymous diseases are described depending on the site but the pathology is the same. The commonest of these are Köhler's disease (tibial tuberosity) and Legg-Calvé-Perthe's disease (head of femur).

442 Osteitis fibrosa cystica, or von Recklinghausen's disease of bone, describes the pathological changes occurring in bone as a result of hyperparathyroidism. Clinically there is bone pain and spontaneous fractures. Grossly the bone is replaced by brown, cystic haemorrhagic tissue. Microscopically there is intense osteoclastic activity, large numbers of these multinucleate giant cells causing resorption of the bone which is then replaced by very vascular fibrous tissue. This may be so prolific as to resemble a giant cell tumour of bone. Haemorrhage from the newly-formed blood vessels occurs with cyst formation. The osteoclastic activity results in hypercalcaemia, metastatic calcification and renal stones.

443 1. A raised alkaline phosphate reflecting osteoblastic activity.
2. A raised urine peptide-bound hydroxyproline reflecting osteoclastic activity.
3. A normal serum calcium and phosphate despite a bone turnover 40–50 times greater than normal.

444 In the early stages there is increased resorptive and regenerative activity in the bone. Resorption is more marked at first and the bone is lighter, fibrosed and has a greatly increased blood supply. Osteoclasts and osteoblasts are prominent. The new bone laid down increases the thickness of both the compact bone and the trabeculae in the spongy bone, and tends to be woven rather than lamellar. The cement lines, which reflect removal

and deposition form a characteristic mosaic pattern. As the disease progresses, the vascularity decreases and the bones become thicker and heavier.

445 Seventy per cent of all bone tumours are metastatic lesions from primary tumours elsewhere, the commonest being from the breast, lung, prostate, kidney and thyroid. With the exception of prostatic secondaries which are osteosclerotic, they are usually osteolytic. Secondary deposits in bone settle first in haemopoietic marrow.

446 1. Tumours of bone tissue:
   a. osteoma and osteoid osteoma; benign tumours
   b. osteogenic sarcoma (osteosarcoma)
2. Tumours of cartilage:
   a. ecchondroma (cartilage capped exostosis) and enchondroma; benign but may become
   b. chondrosarcoma
3. Giant cell tumour of bone (histogenesis doubtful), considered benign but has malignant potential.
4. Tumours of connective and other non-bony tissues:
   a. fibroma (benign) and fibrosarcoma
   b. chordoma
   c. solitary plasmacytoma and multiple myeloma
   d. connective tissue and neural tumours e.g. haemangioma, lipoma and neurofibroma with their malignant counterparts

447 This tumour arises in the medulla of a metaphysis and diaphysis. Arising in the former the epiphyseal cartilage may act as a temporary barrier to tumour spread. The tumour permeates and destroys first the cortex to form a large subperiosteal mass and then the periosteum to infiltrate the surrounding soft tissues. The gross appearance is largely determined by the degree of ossification. Commonly the tumour is vascular with soft necrotic areas interspersed with bone and cartilage. Microscopically it consists of fibrosarcomatous parts formed of spindle cells laying down collagen, chondrosarcomatous areas and poorly differentiated osteoid undergoing calcification and ossification. In some areas osteoclasts may be present where normal bone is being destroyed.

448 This tumour commonly develops in patients between 20 and 40 years of age at the end of a long bone; one half of all tumours occurring at the knee. The tumour is osteolytic, growing slowly and finally elevating the periosteum which then forms a thin shell of normal bone. Because of its osteolytic nature many of these tumours present as pathological fractures. Macroscopically the tumour forms a reddish mass with areas of necrosis. Following penetration of the periosteum infiltration of adjacent soft tissues occurs.

Histologically the tumour is composed of small, fairly uniform cells interspersed with large multinucleate cells resembling osteoclasts. Some tumours are malignant *ab initio* but approximately 50 per cent can be satisfactorily treated by local excision.

Other lesions which have similar appearances and from which this tumour must be distinguished are, osteitis fibrosa cystica, aneurysmal bone cyst and non-ossifying fibroma.

449 This tumour occurs most commonly in young people between 5 and 20 years of age and is highly malignant. The cell of origin remains unknown. It occurs particularly in the long bones and is frequently associated with fever, anaemia and a leucocytosis. It arises in the medullary cavity of long bones and involves both the shaft and the metaphysis. The cortex is soon penetrated causing elevation of the periosteum which responds by laying down layers of new bone, producing the characteristic onion-skin appearance seen on X-ray. Microscopically the tumour is composed of syncytial sheets of small round or polyhedral-shaped cells divided by strands of collagen. A secondary neuroblastoma deposit in bone, having a similar appearance, may be misdiagnosed as a Ewing's tumour.

450 Tumours composed of cartilage arise chiefly in bone but may also arise in cartilage itself or soft tissues.
 1. Benign tumours of cartilage are classified as ecchondromata or enchondromata.
    a. The ecchondroma is also known as osteocartilaginous exostosis or cartilage capped osteoma. It consists of cartilaginous outgrowths which become ossified at their base, from the ends of the long bones. The

growth thus appears to be of bone with a cartilaginous cap although eventually the whole tumour may be converted into well differentiated bone.
   b. Enchondroma—this tumour occurs within the bone. It may be solitary, or multiple when the condition is known as Ollier's disease. Malignancy may supervene in the latter case.
2. Malignant tumours. Unlike osteosarcomata which occur in young people, chondrosarcomata arise in the middle-aged and elderly. They have a wide spectrum of malignancy, highly differentiated tumours being difficult to distinguish from benign chondromata.

451 A chordoma is a tumour derived from the notochordal remnants of the axial skeleton and most commonly occurs in the sacrococcygeal region and the base of the skull. It forms well-circumscribed, lobulated masses greyish in colour, frequently with a gelatinous appearance. Microscopically the tumour consists of lobules of round or polyhedral cells some of which contain intracytoplasmic mucin; the 'physaliferous (bubble-bearing) cells'. Such tumours are slow-growing and usually cause death by local pressure effects.

452 It begins as an acute synovitis, the severity of which is determined by the virulence of the causative organism and host resistance. The joint effusion may be serous, seropurulent or frankly purulent. As the joint fills with pus, proteolytic enzymes released from the polymorphonuclear leucocytes destroy the articular cartilage and underlying bone. The rising intra-articular pressure causes necrosis of soft tissues such as the joint ligaments and capsule so that eventually a sinus may form. If the joint is destroyed, repair usually results in a fibrous ankylosis with the capsule becoming fibrotic, thickened and inelastic.

453 This condition is most commonly caused by *Staphylococcus aureus*, *Streptococcus pyogenes*, *Streptococcus pneumoniae*, *Neisseria gonorrhoeae* and *Salmonella typhi*.

454 The disease begins as synovitis, the synovium becoming hyperaemic, oedematous and swollen. The lining cells proliferate and the underlying

tissue becomes infiltrated with lymphocytes and plasma cells, this inflamed synovium forming the 'pannus'. An auto-immune response to the Fc portion of IgG is believed to be responsible. Immunological complexes from the pannus leak into the joint fluid provoking further inflammation and as the pannus grows across the articular cartilage the latter is destroyed leaving bone exposed. In severe disease, fibrous ankylosis may develop or dislocation of an affected joint may occur, especially in disease affecting the cervical vertebrae or the joints of the fingers respectively.

455 1. Marked hyperplasia of the cortical germinal centres of the lymph nodes.
2. The patient's serum nearly always contains immunoglobulins of the IgM class directed against his IgG.
3. An intense infiltration of the synovial membrane with lymphocytes and plasma cells.
4. A frequent association with systemic lupus erythematosus.
5. The disease is commoner in women than in men.

456 1. Sjögren's syndrome.
2. Polyarteritis nodosa.
3. Psoriasis.
4. Dyshaemopoietic anaemia.

457 Juvenile rheumatoid arthritis. In affected areas bone growth is disorganised resulting in shortening, premature closure of epiphyses, irregularity of shape and dislocation of the joints. The splenomegaly and lymphadenopathy which is considered typical of Still's disease may also occur in adult rheumatoid arthritis.

458 Osteoarthrosis is a common, slowly progressive disease of diarthrodial joints, especially those subjected to excess wear and tear, in which the following pathological changes occur:
1. focal degeneration causing fibrillation and finally loss of the articular cartilage
2. sclerosis of the subchondral bone
3. the development of subchondral cysts at sites of greatest stress
4. the outgrowth of marginal osteophytes
5. increasing deformity of affected joints due to remodelling of articular surfaces

6. the development of loose bodies in affected joints, particularly the knees

459
1. Advancing age.
2. Sex; women being more freqently affected than men.
3. Heredity.
4. Obesity.
5. Incongruity of the articular surfaces which most commonly occurs as a result of fractures involving the joint surfaces.
6. Alterations in skeletal architecture and other causes of excessive and abnormal stresses on the joint.
7. Healed infective arthritis.
8. Healed rheumatoid arthritis.

460
1. Gout caused by the deposition of uric acid in articular cartilage and periarticular tissues.
2. Pseudogout in which pyrophosphate crystals are deposited in the joint cartilage.
3. Alkaptonuria, in which homogentisic acid is deposited, particularly in the intervertebral discs and the articular cartilage of the lips.
4. Hyperparathyroidism, in which osteoclastic proliferation causes periosteal erosions and bone destruction.

461 Haemophilia, a rare bleeding disorder, especially affects the knee joints. Bleeding into the joint occurs spontaneously or within a few minutes of a trivial injury. The blood causes a chronic synovitis and a persistent, painful knee, and with every attack movement of the joint becomes increasingly limited because of capsular thickening. Finally a fibrous or bony ankylosis may develop.

462 This is the result of denervation of the joint and may be caused by multiple sclerosis, diabetic neuropathy, neurosyphilis, leprosy or syringomyelia. Instability together with excessive osteophytic formation is characteristic of this type of joint. A similar joint lesion can occur following repeated intra-articular injection of glucocorticoids.